Love Letters

Restoring Trust While Navigating
the U.S. Healthcare System

to Patients™

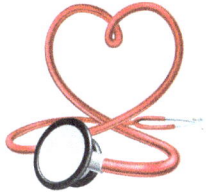

Dr. Ruby J. Long

Emergency Physician & Restorative Justice Expert

LOS ANGELES * LAS VEGAS

LOVE LETTERS TO PATIENTS™
Restoring Trust While Navigating
The U.S. Healthcare System

ISBN   978-1-960001-37-5 (Paperback)
ISBN: 978-1-960001-38-2 (Ebook)
Library of Congress Control Number: 2024906953

Cover/Interior Design: Juan Roberts | Creative Lunacy

KP Publishing Company
Publisher of Fiction, Nonfiction
and Children's Books
www.kp-pub.com

Printed in the United States of America

"Together, you and I, can redefine what good health care is . . . and what good health is."

IMAGE ACKNOWLEDGEMENT

All images in this book are original creations, generated to visually interpret and complement the content. These images are crafted specifically for this project, with no intention to mislead, misrepresent, or mimic any other work. Our aim is to respect and uphold copyright laws, ensuring that each image stands as a unique contribution to the narrative.

DISCLAIMER

Information within this text should not be considered as (personalized) medical advice. Each person using this book should have an evaluation by their medical doctor/provider for medical care and therapy recommendations. Many resources are provided in this book. Consider these resources as a starting point, and they should not be considered all inclusive.

The Love Letters to Patients™ stories and characters of this text are not based on any specific individual, rather a culmination of medical literature. Any similarity to a specific individual or healthcare system is purely coincidental.

CONFLICT OF INTEREST

Views expressed in this text are those informed by my role as an independent restorative justice provider and a medical doctor.

Table of Contents

Dedication

Acknowledgement

Foreword

What Experts Are Saying

Introduction

Chapter 1   Weak & Wobbly

Chapter 2   Heaviness in Your Chest

Chapter 3   Cancer, What!

Activity

Chapter 4   LGBTQ+ Hope in Healthcare? Nope!

Chapter 5   Pregnancy Pains & Precautions

Chapter 6   Tiny Hurts. No, Children Feel Trauma, Too!

Chapter 7   Guns, Guns, Guns ...

Activity

Chapter 8   Overdone By the Overdose

Chapter 9   COVID-19: Is That Still a Thing?

Chapter 10   End of Life is Not the End of Hope

Chapter 11   The Power in Making Your Choices Known

Activity

Chapter 12   RJ as an Rx for Hope

Chapter 13   Helpful Practices When Engaging

the U.S. Healthcare System

Chapter 14   Author's Love Letter of Gratitude to Patients

Chapter 15   Author's Heart-to-Heart Letter to Providers

Chapter 16   Patient Health History

Chapter 17   Resources

The Author

References

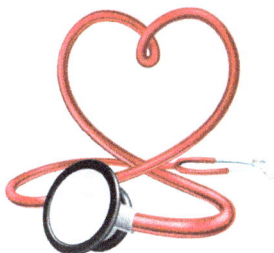

Dedication

To the greatest love of my life, my son, DJ. You have taught me how to be present in this moment and to unleash the power of my words. You teach me endless compassion for every kind soul. Thank you for giving me the courage of a mama bear to be brave when the time calls.

—Mama loves you, DJ

Acknowledgement

I am thankful for the wisdom and healing that started at family tables. To the pioneers of healing known and unknown, thank you for sharing your knowledge. I humbly pay respect to the past and present elders of the lands that founded the United States for their resilience to LIVE against colonization. Most explicitly, thank you, Dr. Rebecca Lee Crumpler, Ms. Ella Baker and Mrs. Fannie Lou Hamer, for sacrificing your time, energy and bodies for the advancement of human rights. Mrs. Assilene Ezell Long, thank you for always cheering for me and brushing me off after a fall.

Foreword

Dr. Ruby Long's book, **Love Letters to Patients™,** is a beacon of hope and empowerment in the often complex landscape of the U.S. healthcare system. As a Physician Leader and Health Equity Advocate, Dr. Long draws on her extensive experience as a patient, medical professional and advocate to address the widening healthcare disparities in the United States.

The book serves as an invaluable tool. The collection of letters resonates with patients and their supporters, offering comfort and guidance during moments of uncertainty and fear. With a keen focus on marginalized communities, Dr. Long emphasizes the importance of equitable healthcare and treatment, empowering those who often feel unheard by the healthcare system.

Love Letters to Patients goes beyond a mere guide; it is a testament to Dr. Long's dedication to restoring trust in healthcare. The top ten causes of death and harm are presented as patient-centered, offering practical information, evidence-based treatment options, and self-advocacy tips. The book covers a range of crucial topics, from heart attacks and strokes to LGBTQ+ affirming care, with a particular emphasis on under-resourced communities.

This book is not just a source of information but a source of inspiration, reminding readers that they have the right to ask questions and voice concerns about their healthcare. Dr. Ruby Long's compassionate approach, drawn from her own experiences and two decades in healthcare, ensures that ***Love Letters to Patients*** is a powerful tool for anyone navigating medical episodes.

In conclusion, ***Love Letters to Patients*** is a heartfelt and impactful contribution that will undoubtedly make a difference in the lives of those seeking understanding, support, and empowerment within the healthcare system. Dr. Ruby Long's dedication to restoring trust and advocating for health equity shines through every page of this invaluable guide. I am grateful for this perspective and trust you will be, too!

—Barbara A. Perkins
Executive Coach and
Community Advocate

What Experts Are Saying...

In Love Letters to Patients: Restoring Trust While Navigating the U.S. Healthcare System, Dr. Ruby J. Long expertly merges her vast healthcare experience with a profound empathy for patients. This groundbreaking book is an essential tool for anyone in the healthcare field, emphasizing the importance of patient-centered care and the role of healthcare professionals in advocating for patients. Dr. Long's innovative approach to addressing healthcare disparities through personal letters offers practical guidance and a compassionate perspective, making it a beacon for enhancing patient-provider relationships and advancing healthcare equity. Her work is a testament to the power of understanding and empathy in transforming healthcare.

—**Arica Brandford**, RN, JD, PhD

Love Letters to Patients, curated and written with devotion and fierceness by Dr. Ruby Long, demonstrates the capacity and responsibility individuals within oppressive systems have to re-humanize, and even to re-spiritualize, the tender spaces within our society where we care for our most vulnerable. It is not only evidenced through the content of this work but also by the format, which seeks to gently, yet firmly, provide clinicians and patients with an accessible blueprint for effective and humanistic care.

Dr. Long uses her own life, intersections and, experiences to highlight the cracks in healthcare and provides us with language and practices to remove the band-aids and finally care for the deep wounds within. *Love Letters To Patients* is a gift to us all: providers, patients and, if they will dare to change, policy-makers."

—Thea Monyeé
Founder of MarleyAyo Inc. and
The Blacker The Brain Collective

Dr. Ruby Long's book, Love Letters to Patients: Restoring Trust While Navigating the U.S. Healthcare System, is an invaluable gem that resonates deeply with healthcare professionals like myself. As a nurse, I wholeheartedly appreciate Dr. Long's dedication to shedding light on the pervasive health disparities within our healthcare system.

Her insightful exploration of crucial topics including heart disease, cancer, pregnancy, substance abuse, and end-of-life care reflects a profound understanding of the challenges faced by marginalized individuals in accessing quality healthcare based on her personal experience as an Emergency Room Physician.

Dr. Long's compassionate approach not only enlightens but also empowers both patients and healthcare providers alike. Her unique blend of professional expertise and compassionate storytelling not only educates but also inspires. By drawing upon her own experiences, she provides invaluable insights and practical guidance for navigating the complexities of our healthcare landscape. **Love Letters to Patients** is more than just a book;

it's a testament to Dr. Long's unwavering commitment to healing and advocacy.

Through her eloquent prose, she fosters a sense of empathy and understanding, while empowering patients to embrace their agency in their healthcare journey.

—**Nikki Taylor**, RN, BSN, MSN, AGCNS

Introduction

This book will serve as a way to bring up questions and concerns when things feel scary and out of control during a medical event. Enclosed you will find a collection of letters filled with hope and empowerment to patients/patient supporters from a Physician Leader and Health Equity Advocate. Common conditions that cause the most harm to health and life are presented in these letters. Readers will be aware of how these conditions show up as symptoms in the real world, be informed of the best science-based treatments, and gain self-advocacy tips during unsettling times.

This book will open up conversations about the American health system's layout and service delivery. To get the most out of this book, look at the table of contents to see what piques your interest. Then, flip through the book to absorb the images of respectful healthcare. Next, you can read the book by section of interest to you or from cover to cover. Start at any place that speaks to you. Just start. Consider reading Chapter 13, Helpful Practices When Engaging the U.S. Healthcare System, before practicing the techniques in this book. If you want more information about a topic, references are in parenthesis at the end of sentences. Details of each reference are listed at the back of the book. If you need more clarity, please email our support team at support@loveletterstopatients.org. **Love Letters To Patients**™ will show examples of restorative justice in action, and its use as a tool to support and grow healing. This book will deepen your understanding of the tiers of Restorative Justice and empower you with advocacy tools for local implementation.

Together, you and I can redefine what good healthcare is and what good health is. Proceeds from this book will support organizations' doing just work to close healthcare gaps of marginalized communities within the United States.

May each day of life bring moments of joy and empowerment. Your tears and hurts are not in vain.

With love, the *Casualty Doc*®,

Dr. Ruby J. Long

Dr. Ruby J. Long

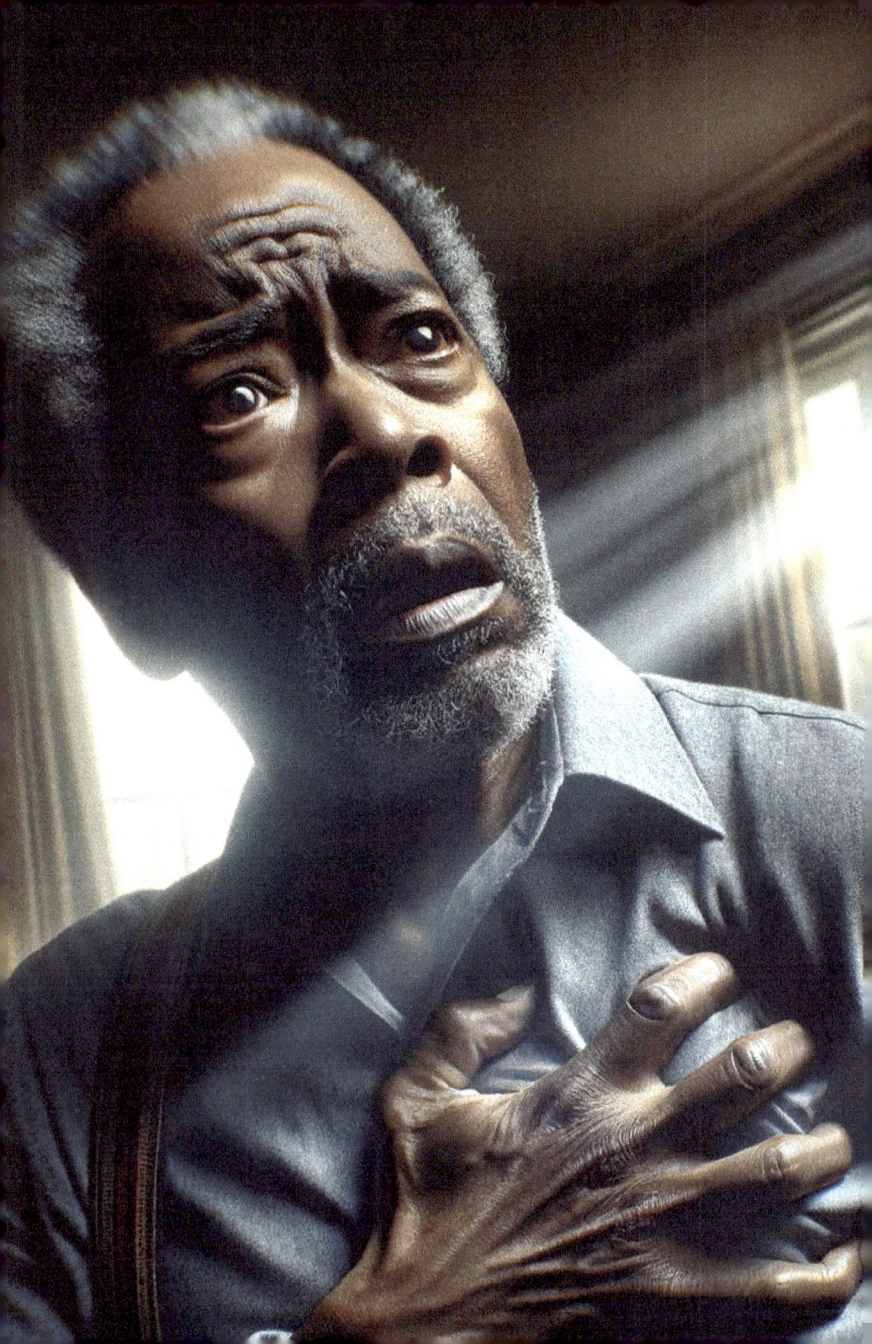

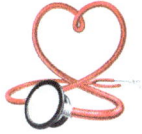

Chapter 1

Weak & Wobbly
STROKE

Compassionate Letter

My precious, I understand you were preparing to wind down for the evening. You amazed yourself this time with how many things you could get done in one day. Towards the end of dinner, you noticed that it seemed a little difficult to get your cup to your mouth. You downplayed the dribble from the side of your face when you drank. You thought you were just moving too fast.

You decided that you needed to relax and figured that you would make this an early night and head to bed. Your sleep was restless for most of the night. You awoke in a daze. When you really started to move about, the inability to talk and move your arm was too real. Your mind was in overdrive. I'm so glad that your other hand could dial 9-1-1, and you could open the door for the rescue squad.

Now here at the hospital, I must tell you that you had a major stroke. Our team will hurry to see if this is a bleeding stroke or a clot stroke. You are our most valuable patient at this moment. This is what we train for. We will jump into our highest performance mode: scans, monitors, labs, and EKGs (electrocardiograms/electric tracings of the heart from stickers on your chest). The outcome of these tests will guide the treatment you will receive. Yes, I understand that so much is happening fast. Once we get the scans, we can slow down and talk about all your options for care. Getting answers for you is everyone's top goal right now.

The scans didn't take very long, and we were with you every step of the way. The tests confirm that you had a large ischemic stroke due to cholesterol and a debris clot that got lodged in part of your brain's artery. Our hands are tied with the treatment we can offer. Too much time has passed for us to give you the clot buster medication (thrombolytics/tPA) to dissolve that clot (AHA T). The risks of the side effects, of major bleeding, only grow with time. Our main goal is to "do no harm" per the Hippocratic Oath. We can do one more test to see if the clot that formed the stroke is large enough to be seen with a special dye. Occasionally, the Stroke Team can use their tools in the cath lab to pull out the clot or dissolve it with a small dose of the clot buster medication right where the artery is blocked (AHA T). What questions do you have?

I understand the fear and frustration you have. Will you sound like this forever? Will you be able to hold your grandchild without dropping them? And what about sex? Right now, try your best to relax. We need to keep your blood pressure under good control. Increased stress can elevate your blood pressure and possibly make the stroke worse. Our team is smart and kind. We are dedicated to working with you every step of the way to get your strength back and your hopes up. Everyone in the Neuro wing has special training which improves the chances for stroke patients to get back to their daily activities independently. I know this is overwhelming. Try to take it day by day, moment by moment.

Down to Earth explanation

Strokes are a form of cardiovascular disease. This is a disease of the blood vessels that lead to and from the heart. It is all too common. Strokes are the fifth most common cause of death in the United States.

Strokes are a significant cause of people losing control of bodily processes and movements which contribute to disability.

There are two major types of strokes. Stroke from clots that reduce blood flow to the brain make up the bulk of strokes in the United States (U.S.). This is also known as an ischemic stroke. The other type of stroke is the hemorrhagic stroke. That occurs when the arteries that carry blood inside the brain open up and lead to uncontrolled bleeding and pressure on the brain. Both types of strokes show up similarly in the function of our bodies. They both rob people of routine movement, speech, thinking, and other bodily functions. Time is the most precious resource during a stroke scenario. Every minute of a stroke can cause permanent damage to the brain. There are also certain time frames to safely give stroke reversing medications without causing more harm to stroke patients.

My Dear, do not put off going to the hospital to see if you get better on your own. One hour is even too much time to delay stroke care. Go to the closest hospital available to you as soon as you notice something is not right. Do not downplay symptoms that come and go for a few minutes at a time. You might notices symptoms that come in waves of less than 5 minutes (AHA TIA). Those are signs of "mini-strokes" also known as TIAs (transient ischemic attacks). Mini (mini-stroke) is actually a mighty force warning you that a major stroke is on the horizon. Usually within three months of a mini-stroke, 18% of people will have a major stroke if the mini-stroke is not cared for (AHA S). Actually, Mini is quite impatient, half of the people in that 18% figure will have a major stroke within two days of Mini showing up.

Care Considerations

Stroke treatment options are geared towards restoring normal blood flow in the brain and minimizing the risk of recurrence. The sooner you can access treatment, the lower the chance of long-lasting damage or death from a stroke (AHA T). Depending on the cause of the stroke, medications (e.g., thrombolytics), surgery, and/or high blood pressure medications (e.g., anti-hypertensives) may be necessary to help regain brain function. Even if your neighborhood hospital is not a "Certified Stroke Center" or teaching hospital, there should be protocols in place to start stroke care and escalate as needed to specialty centers to ensure patients get the best stroke care possible. Not wasting time in the treatment of new strokes is very important. Get to the closest hospital possible.

U.S. Quick Facts

Stroke

U.S. OVERVIEW

- **Ranking as Cause of Death:**
#5 in the U.S. (CDC FastStats)
- **Nature:** Immediate loss of partial brain function due to abnormal blood flow.
- **Impact:** Stroke is a significant cause of disability in the U.S.

Pearls for Further Explanation

Act F.A.S.T.:
- **F**ace drooping
- **A**rms difficulty
- **S**peech slurring
- **T**ime to call 911

- **Call 9-1-1 right away** if you or someone you are with shows any signs of a stroke (CDC Stroke). **Llame 9-1-1**.

• **Urgency:** Prompt action is crucial in stroke scenarios. Delay can lead to death or severe disability.

• **Preventability:** Up to 80% of strokes can be prevented.

• Time is the greatest factor in reducing death and permanent disability from stroke (AHA T). Get treatment right away.

• Up to 80% of strokes are preventable. Most strokes don't have to happen. (AHA Stroke).

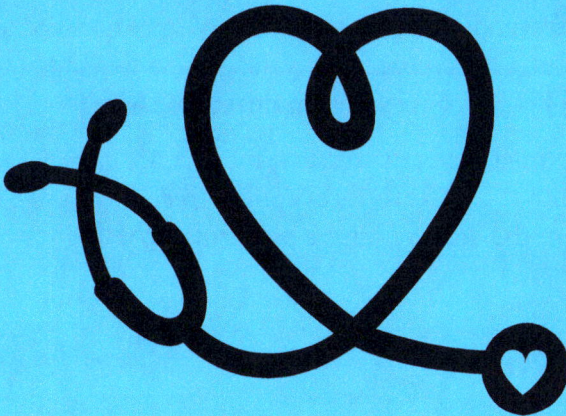

Types of Strokes

ISCHEMIC STROKE
(Clot Stroke)

• 85% of all strokes are the ischemic type (AHA T).

• This is the most common type of stroke health care providers see.

TREATMENTS:

• Optimal blood pressure control, thrombolytics (clot busting medication) or clot retrieval procedures are common treatments.

• Thrombolytics are only available through an IV (intravenously) within 3 hours of stroke symptom onset. On rare occasions this can be expanded to 4.5 hours from symptom onset (AHA T).

• In really select cases that meet strict criteria, endovascular care (procedures to remove the clot from the artery) can be performed (AHA T).

HEMORRHAGIC STROKE
(Bleeding Stroke)

Bleeding from an artery (or arteries) of the brain makes up a small portion of all strokes.

TREATMENTS:
• Optimal blood pressure control.
• Reversal agents or antidotes to counteract certain blood thinners.
• Invasive procedures or surgeries are the primary treatment tools for Hemorrhagic Stroke.

TIA (Transient Ischemic Attack)
(Mini Stroke)

• TIAs are due to a temporary blockage of an artery in the brain from a clot (AHA Stroke).

• TIAs can mimic a stroke for a duration of a few minutes up to 24 hours (AHA Stroke).

• TIAs are a warning sign that patients are at risk of a major stroke soon (AHA TIA).

Pearls for Further Explanation

• Almost 33% "of people who have a TIA, have a major stroke within one year (AHA TIA)."

• TIAs and strokes cause the same symptoms at the beginning. It is impossible to tell them apart at the start, so get to the hospital right away (AHA TIA).

RX FOR SELF-ADVOCACY

Questions to ask with
Weak & Wobbly Stroke Symptoms

• Did I have a mini-stroke (Transient Ischemic Attack (TIA)) or a massive stroke?

• Do I qualify for clot busters (thrombolytics) or any procedure to get the clot from the artery in my brain?

• What can I do to prevent this from happening again?

Didn't I See That in the News?

Mr. Luther Vandross

When Mr. Luther Vandross opened his mouth, the world was in for a treat. It was time to get close to the one you loved and groove to his velvety voice. His stage presence almost topped his voice, but it was never too much. This dapper singer-song writer never again had that same energy after his stroke in May 2003.

The initial stroke kept Mr. Vandross in a coma for two months after it occurred. He was never able to walk by himself again. Just two years from the stroke, Mr. Luther Vandross died unexpectedly on July 1, 2005 (Garrett). It was so amazing that Luther Vandross died at a youthful 54-years-old (Garrett) from complications of his stroke and cardiovascular disease. It is hoped that he truly understood how much he was loved.

"Luther, may your dance never end. You have given us a soundtrack to unconditional love."

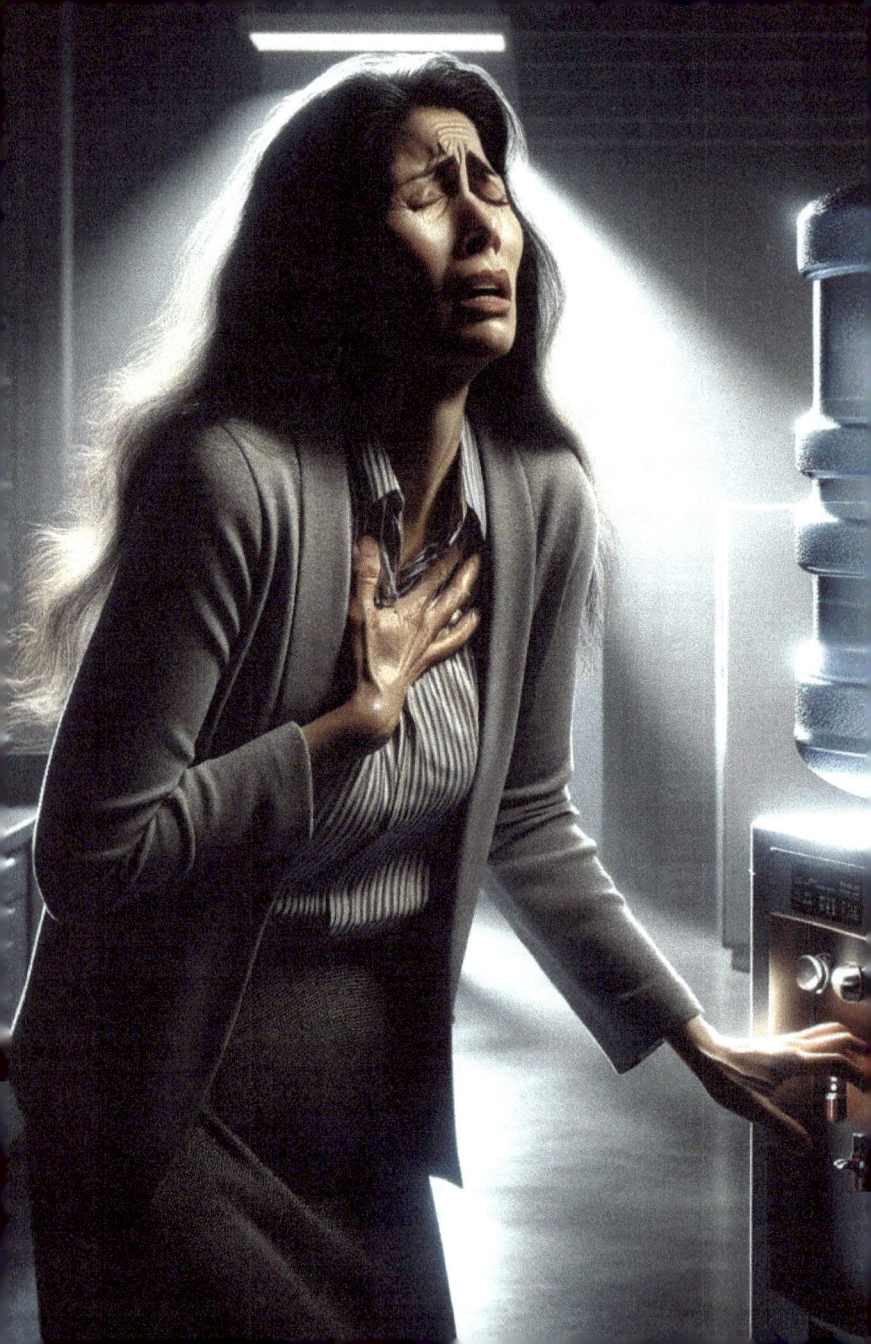

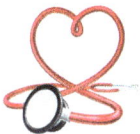

Chapter 2

Heaviness in Your Chest
CHEST DISCOMFORT

Compassionate Letter

Oh my dear, that feeling of heaviness in your chest is not to be dismissed. The ache grabbed you as you got dressed to start your day. You were certain that you pulled a muscle. Then you shrugged it off to get to work. I totally understand that the bills won't pay themselves.

School drop-offs done. Neither of the kids forgot anything at home. You took the back way into the job to dodge traffic. When you slid into your desk chair, you could finally take a deep breath and have a moment to relax before the office drama began.

You knew something wasn't right when your neck and jaw began to feel tight with pressure. It wasn't the financial forecast that was being presented during the meeting, and it wasn't the boxed lunch. I'm so thankful that when you got up to get coffee, someone noticed that you didn't look right and said that you should get checked out. You made a note in your head and thought: "I'll go right after work. It's busy season at the job. I can't take time away from work now."

As the day went on, you noticed that it was harder and harder to get from your desk to the restroom. You thought if you just breathed a little harder, you'd be okay. Your co-workers knew that look in your eyes and called 9-1-1. Now you and I meet, and I must tell you that you are having a heart attack. The Cath Lab and the Heart Team are waiting to care for you.

My Dear, no, this is not tension from the busy season at work! And no, you are not crazy! I know this is scary and getting you to the Cath Lab is the best next step to keep you from dying. Blood is not flowing to your heart like normal. This can't go on much longer before permanent damage or death comes.

I checked on you later, and you said that you got a stent in your heart. I'm so thankful to hear your voice. You are one of the lucky ones. Many don't live to tell their story.

Down to Earth explanation

Cardiovascular (Heart & Vessel) Disease is the number one cause of death in the U.S. Heart attacks make up the majority of the deaths from cardiovascular disease. This disease occurs as cholesterol and debris (e.g., plaque) build up in arteries over time. This buildup of plaque can happen all over the body. Most commonly, the plaque builds to the point that it cuts off blood flow or a piece breaks off, reducing blood flow. When this blockage occurs in the heart, it causes a heart attack (AHA Heart). Occasionally, the arteries
that move blood to the heart spasm (tense up) or the layers of the arteries separate from one another (a.k.a. dissection) causing a heart attack (AHA Heart). Every 40 seconds, someone has a heart attack in the U.S. (AHA Heart).

Care Considerations

Heart attack treatment goals are to restore normal blood flow to the heart as soon as possible. Every minute of an untreated heart attack can lead to serious damage (AHA Heart) which may not be reversible. Medications (e.g., aspirin or heparin) make it easier for blood to flow through an injured heart. Procedures, such as heart cath (catheterization) or coronary artery bypass graft (CABG, pronounced cabbage) surgery are often used to save lives during a massive heart attack.

U.S. Quick Facts

Heart Disease

• **#1 cause of death in the U.S.** is heart disease.

• **The risk of heart disease** increases in the presence of other medical conditions like diabetes, obesity, excessive alcohol use, and lack of physical exercise (CDC Heart Disease).

Pearls for Further Explanation

• **The Million Hearts Campaign** has sharable videos you can post on social media.

• **Move More for a Healthy Heart** – explains how physical activity can have a positive impact on your heart.

• **Keep Your Cholesterol in Check** – explains the impact healthy eating can have on controlling your cholesterol (Million Hearts).

Heart Attack

• Just about every minute of the day, someone has a heart attack in this country. Actually, "every 40 seconds" a heart attack is recorded (AHA Heart, CDC Heart).

• **Silent Heart Attacks** are dangerous because they make up 20% of all heart attacks (CDC Heart). Folks often notice that they just don't have energy, have terrible indigestion (AHA Heart), or shortness of breath with a silent heart attack.

• **Women** are at "a 20% increased risk of developing heart failure or dying within five years after their first severe heart attack compared with men" (AHA Newsroom).

• **Time to treatment** for heart attack determines the amount of damage (AHA Heart Attack).

• **Evidence-Based Therapies** often mentioned are: Aspirin, Heparin, Thrombolytics, Nitroglycerin, Heart Catheterization, Coronary Artery Bypass Graft Surgery (CABG).

Resources

- **Call 1-800-AHA-USA1 (1-800-242-8721)** or visit heart.org for a deeper look at heart disease and stroke (AHA What is a Heart).

- **AHA Heart Attack Tip Sheet link** (https://www.heart.org/-/media/Files/Health-Topics/Answers-by-Heart/What-is-a-Heart-Attack.pdf)

Heart Failure

• Develops over time because the heart can no longer pump at peak performance (HF). The decline in the heart's pump function limits the amount of blood that flows through our bodies to give us energy.

• Disease to the heart's arteries, high blood pressure and prior heart attacks (HF) commonly cause heart failure in the U.S.

• Symptoms of heart failure can show up as feeling run down (fatigue), shortness of breath, really winded with slight movement, swollen tight legs, sudden weight gain and/or confusion.

• Options for Heart Failure care include specialized medications (HF Meds), lifestyle changes (AHA What is HF), small medical heart devices (AICDs or LVADs), or catheter-based procedures to improve blood flow (HFDevices).

Resources

• **AHA What is HF link** https://www.heart.org/en/health-topics/heart-failure/what-is-heart-failure

RX FOR SELF-ADVOCACY

Questions to Ask With Heaviness In Your Chest/Chest Discomfort Symptoms:

• What did my EKG (electrocardiogram—traces electrical activity of your heart) show? Did it show a heart attack?

• What were my troponins (heart marker proteins), normal or high? Did the troponins show that I had a mild (or silent) heart attack.?

• For heart failure, know your EF (ejection fraction) and ask what treatments are available to you at each % (percentage) EF.

Didn't I See That in the News?

Mr. Kamakawiwo'ole was also known as "Iz®" by many who loved him. He made a career from delivering hope for a his brighter future with his soothing voice, gentle presence and his ukulele. His voice stopped people in their tracks. Then his energy made people feel good, safe, and happy when he sang (Iz® Bio). As a son of Hawaii, Iz embodied the aloha spirit (UH). He had great respect for the ways of the elders and concern for the people and the islands. He hoped to support all on the islands in building respectful community with one another and the land. He was an advocate for humanity (Enomoto). He understood that his time on Earth would be temporary and providing protection/stability for those he loved was key (Montagne).

It was uncertain if Bruddah Iz innately knew that he would not have a physical life of longevity on this Earth, or if he was just taking a wide-eyed view to his family trends (Montagne). Both of his parents died young at age 47 and 55 from heart disease. Iz's older brother died at age 27 from heart attack, and his younger sister died at age 21. Shortly after Iz's 30th birthday (and releasing his Grammy Award® winning album), he had his first heart attack (NPR Iz®). Ultimately, Iz died at 38 years old from complications of his cardiovascular disease (Montagne). Mr. Kamakawiwo'ole, your wonderful smile of hope warms our souls from somewhere over the rainbow.

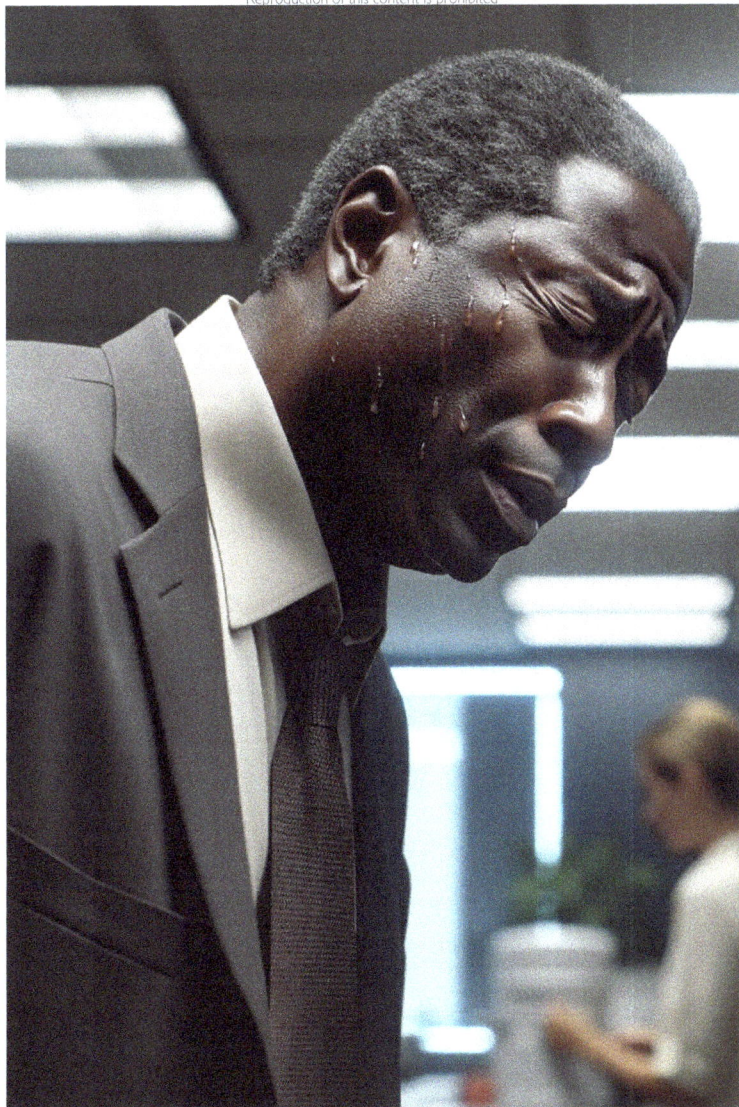

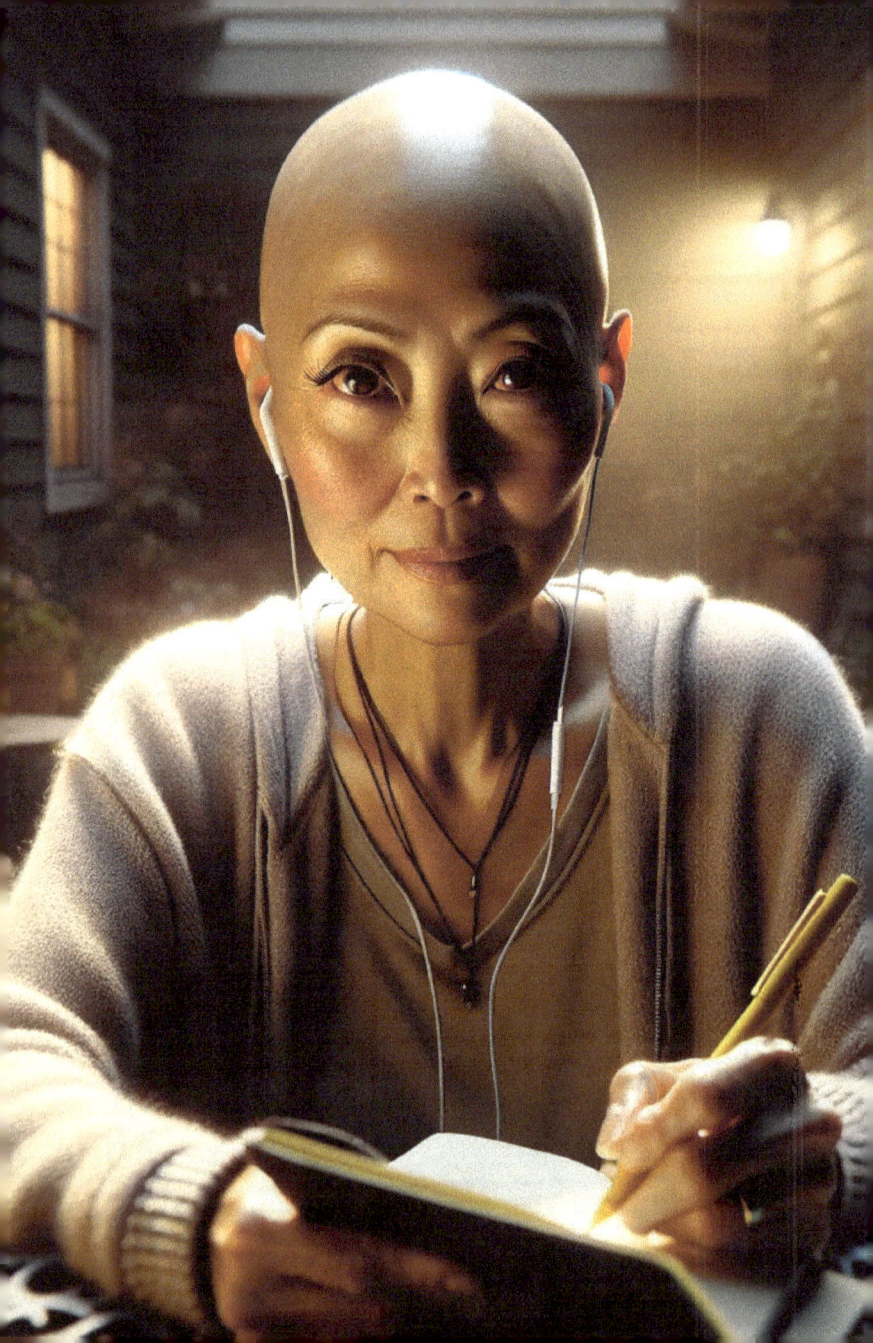

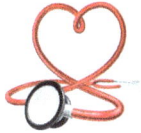

Chapter 3

Cancer, What?!

Compassionate Letter

Kindred, of course you are gorgeous. Yes, I understand that your hair has fallen out and your weight is down. I can still see the brightness of your soul through your eyes. That sparkle in your eyes tells me how wonderful you are. Yes, I know you are strong. You have to be to face this challenge head on as you are. I know it hurts you that you don't run two miles a day then head to the office anymore. Have you thought of walking for just 5-10 minutes each day? Try your best not to worry too much. You know you put your team in a good place prior to leaving the office.

Yes, I understand it's hard to stay focused. The chemo brain fog can be thicker than smog (ACS B). Let's take a deep breath. Umm, how about another? Here's a journal. Write down the things that worry you, and we can talk about them. The tingles in your fingers, they come and go in waves, making it hard to hold the pen. I understand. Many people get those hand-foot neuropathy tingles from the chemo (ACS Non, Alberta). Let's talk to your Cancer Team to see if cool packs can reduce the side effects of the chemo on your nerves. Did you know they even make cooling caps to reduce the amount of hair loss from chemo? Those caps have nothing on your stylish hats.

You are most welcome. It was only IV (intravenous) hydration and medicine for nausea that we gave you. It feels good to hear you say you feel better. Oh wow, your smile now mirrors the sparkle in your eyes. How can you hold on to that tiny joy? Try each day to find a moment of joy. Even if it's just to know that you woke up this day or that the birds still chirp.

Have you talked to your loves about what is important to you? Have you started to dream about life after cancer? You must hold on to the hope that there will be life after cancer. It's the hope that will get you through. Do you have help to get food, make your appointments, or clean your clothes? Is there anything we can do today to lighten the load for you?

Down to Earth explanation

Cancer is the second leading cause of death in the United States (Ahmad). Disease from cancer is caused by uncontrolled growth of the cells in the body (NCI). Every system of the body is made up of a collection of cells. When a collection of cells are in sync, we see that as an organ (e.g., skin, lungs, kidneys). When the cells are no longer in sync or getting the correct signals because the programing from the control center (i.e., our genes) has been damaged, the cancer cells result. The cancerous cells over-grow and invade organs and surrounding tissues. More than 100 different types of cancer exist (NCI). The cancers are typically named according to "the organs or tissues where the cancers form (NCI)." Thus, cancers that start on the skin are called skin cancers. When the cancerous cells spread any distance from the original cancer cell cluster, this is known as metastasis (NCI). Cancer is ranked at different stages (I-IV) based on the location of the cancer, the amount of spread and the appearance of the cells (ACS Staging). Stage I cancers are less advanced and have more treatment options (ACS Staging). As cancers become more complex, the cancer stage number grows (II-IV) and treatment options vary (ACS Staging).

Care Considerations

Cancer treatment and outcomes depend on multiple things. The **patient's wishes**, their age, location of the cancer, time of detection, and available medications or procedures all factor into someone's ability to survive cancer. Medical providers strongly consider the current stage of a cancer when forming a prognosis or outlook for plan of care (ACS Staging).

Many people are familiar with chemotherapy. This is a cocktail of medications to target and fight cancerous cells. Each cancer has a unique response to the chemotherapy agents. Sometimes the chemotherapy can eliminate the cancer all together or slow the cancer down to the point that the person with cancer is still able to live and enjoy life. Certain cancers may respond to reprogramming through gene therapy (Cross, Mckie). Other times, our cells' command centers (i.e., genes) can be reprogramed to help chemotherapy work better (NIH Gene Tx). Depending on the situation, there may be a role for radiation at some point in the journey. Treating teams often engage multiple tools to help with pain control, anxiousness and depression based on patient needs and wishes. True healing is holistic, inclusive of the mind, body and soul.

"You never know how strong you are until being strong is your only choice." —Bob Marley

U.S. Quick Facts

Cancer

• Cancer is the #2 Cause of Death in U.S. (CDC Fast Facts).

• Uncontrolled growth of cells in the body causes cancer (NCI).

• 1 in 3 in the U.S. "will have cancer in their lifetime" (NCCDP HP).

• Up to half of all cases of cancer are preventable, 30-50% according to WHO (WHO Preven CA).

• **Early detection** and prompt treatment improve the cure rate and chance of survival from cancer (WHO Cancer).

• **Regular health exams** with screenings are the key to finding and treating cancer early (WHO).

Resources

American Cancer Society
Cancer Helpline
800.227.2345

"One-on-One Support, Information and Hope available every moment of every day. You don't have to face a cancer diagnosis alone. Talk or chat live with a trained cancer information specialist or find support in your own community."
Call: 1-800-227-2345
https://www.cancer.org

ACS: Helping Children When a Family Member or Someone They Know Has Cancer
https://www.cancer.org/treatment/children-and-cancer/when-a-family-member-has-cancer.html

Skin Cancer

• **#1 cause** of U.S. cancer (CDC Kinds of Cancer)

• **Everyone is at risk** of getting skin cancer, no matter your skin hue.

• **Skin cancer** is often diagnosed at an advanced stage in the skin of people of color (AAD).

• **Over-exposure** to the ultraviolet (UV) light from the sun, tanning booths, and sun lamps lead to most skin cancers.

• **Even on a cloudy day**, the UV rays can reach your skin. UV rays can bounce off water, snow, sand and cement during reflection (CDC Sun Safety).

• **Inspect ALL** of your skin, scalp, finger and toenails, palms and soles at least monthly (AAD).

• **Tricks for protecting your skin from the sun damage:**

- Sit under shade coverings when possible.

- Wear lightweight clothing to cover all of your arms and legs from the sun.

- Wear hats or sunglasses (CDC Sun).

- Use sunblock/ sunscreen that is SPF 30 or higher (AAD).

Breast Cancer

- **#2 cause** of cancer in the U.S. (NCI Common)

- **Men get breast cancer, too** (NCI Common Cancer).

- **People diagnosed** at early stages of breast cancer have a really good chance for cure (Mayo).

Men should be alert for signs of breast cancer in themselves:

- A painless lump in your pec (pectoral) or breast region.

- Skin changes to your pec or breast "such as dimpling, puckering, redness or scaling."

- Your nipples become red, turn inward, scale, or have fluid from the nipple (Mayo).

Lung Cancer

- **#1 cause** of cancer death in the U.S. (CDC).

- **Smoking tobacco** causes 90% of lung cancer.

• Radon, a radioactive gas in the soil, is the second most common cause of lung cancer.

• Cigarette smoke plus Radon increases lung cancer risks even more (ALA).

• "Tobacco smoke has more than 7,000 chemicals; at least 250 are known to be harmful and at least 69 are known to cause cancer" (WHO Prev).

FEMALES*

The most common types of cancer in women are: Breast, bowel (colorectal), "lung, cervical and thyroid cancer" (WHO Cancer).

Breast Cancer

• Become familiar with how your breasts normally look and feel. This will allow you to detect changes and seek care right away, if your breasts change (ACS D).

• Routine mammograms begin at age 40 (Aubrey, ACOG Mamm). These are specialized x-rays that look for cancer cells in breast tissue. Please look at the people in your family for early onset cancers, and let your doctors know (Aubrey).

Cervical Cancer

• **Cervical cancer screening** should occur between 21–25 years of age (ACOG Cerv, ACS D). If you are high risk because of prenatal exposure to toxins, immunocompromised from HIV (ACOG Cervical CA) or smoke tobacco (ACS Cervical Risks), please let your healthcare provider know.

Colon Cancer

• **At 45 years old,** people with average risk for colorectal cancer should start screenings (ACS early Detection).

Lung Cancer

• **Start screening at age 50** if you smoke currently or quit within the last 15 years and have at least 20 packed years of smoking (ACS D).

MALES*

• The most common types of cancer in men are: Lung, Prostate, Bowel (colorectal), Liver and Stomach cancer (WHO Cancer).

Lung Cancer

• **Start screening at age 50** if you smoke currently or quit within the last 15 years and have at least 20 packed years of smoking (ACS D, ACS S).

Prostate Cancer

• **Start regular screening at age 50** if you have average risk.

• **Start screening at 45** or younger if you are African-American or have a father or brother diagnosed with prostate cancer younger than 65 years old (ACS Pro).

Colon Cancer

• **Screening begins at age 45** for people with average risk (ACS D). Please look at the people in your family for early onset cancers and let your healthcare provider know this history. You may need to start screening earlier.

Caregivers of Loved Ones With Cancer

• Seeing your loved one struggle with an illness is taxing.

• Remember to see the world and the cancer through the eyes of your loved one.

• Always be respectful of what your loved one wishes.

• Take care of yourself and take breaks when needed.

Resources for Caregiver Support

• How to talk to your loved one about cancer
• How to talk to the Cancer Treatment Team
• How to care for yourself call:

Call American Cancer Society at 1-800-227-2345 to find respite services in your area (https://www.cancer.org/cancer/caregivers/caregiver-resource-guide.html)

* Current recommendations are based on available data that corresponds to the organs people were born with at birth and the assigned sex of male or female. There is a movement within the scientific community to be more inclusive of transgender and non-binary people (Braun, Jackson, Sterling).

No matter how you express your gender and love for others, be mindful of your internal organs and perform routine screenings as indicated.

RX FOR SELF-ADVOCACY

Questions to ask with Cancer Care:

• What screenings are necessary at my age to detect cancers early when more treatment options exist?

• What can I do to reduce my risk of cancer?

• How do I reduce the side effects of chemo (chemotherapy)?

• What support services are available (e.g., meal delivery, laundry, appointment transportation)?

• How do I tell my family that I have fought as long as I could? What should I do, if I don't want to keep going? How do I tell my family that I am not giving up? Rather the treatments don't leave me with energy to do the things I want?

• How do I find control when everything seems out of control?

Didn't I See That in the News?

Supreme Court Justice
Ruth Bader Ginsburg

Her petite stature made a grand presence on the world. Justice Ginsburg realized that she had a special weapon in her arsenal: her brain. She brilliantly crafted legislation that favored equity and forever changed the way the U.S. sees women, pays women, and provides family rights (Roberts). She used her words to advocate for gender equality and showed how it benefited all people. She literally set the bar for gender equity before her Supreme Court Justice days.

As a practicing attorney and law professor, Ruth Bader Ginsburg had the insight to break down antebellum practices of defaulting to men to manage business affairs over women. "She knew what it was to feel like a second-class citizen" and to be discriminated against for being a woman (Cohen), getting pregnant (Totenberg) and for being a mother that worked outside of the home (Perkins). Her Reed v. Reed brief disrupted a centuries-long standing of presuming that men were innately more capable to manage business affairs than women (Adler). Her work literally became the model that others followed. Justice Ginsburg knew and shared that "real change happens one step at a time" during her Supreme Court Confirmation (Cohen). She transformed outrage into righteousness within the law. Justice Ginsburg showed the world and legislators the real-world impact of how gender-based discrimination hurt everyone (Oyez).

Though she did not see eye to eye with her peers when she dissented, she always kept a respectable working relationship with them. Justice Ginsburg disagreed with ideas and never the person that carried them. She never lost sight of the people the law touched.

Often noted for her "Super Diva" apparel, Justice Ginsburg was never nasty or one to shy away from a good fight. She took this fighting spirit with her in her personal life. Justice Ginsburg found a way to shine and be an academic star among the top of her Harvard Law class as exemplified by her well-earned Law Review position. Amongst the nearly 500 men and 8 other women in her class, she showed them all why she had earned the right to take a seat at the institution (Totenberg). When life threw her curve balls, she dug deep, slept little and got things done. Justice Bader Ginsberg survived multiple bouts of cancer (Totenberg). Cervical cancer took her mother from her when the young Justice Ginsberg (RBG) was just shy of high school graduation (Cohen, Totenberg, Fernald). Cancer struck again while she and her husband, Marty, were young parents and law students at Harvard. Marty survived his grueling testicular cancer journey.

Then, almost 50 years later, Marty took leave of this life (Cohen, Schild) after his battle with metastatic cancer (Perkins). RBG knew cancer intimately from her own personal battles with it, as well. The fifth resurgence of her cancer took Justice Ruth Bader Ginsburg from this life (Totenberg).

Rest in power, Notorious R.B.G! Supreme Court Justice Ruth Bader Ginsburg embodied the American Dream of blazing your own path and changing the future for the better. Thank you for showing us how to take up the space we have earned.

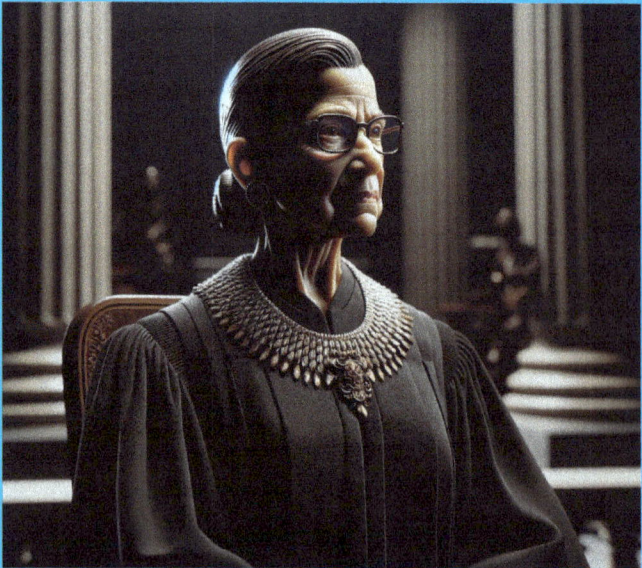

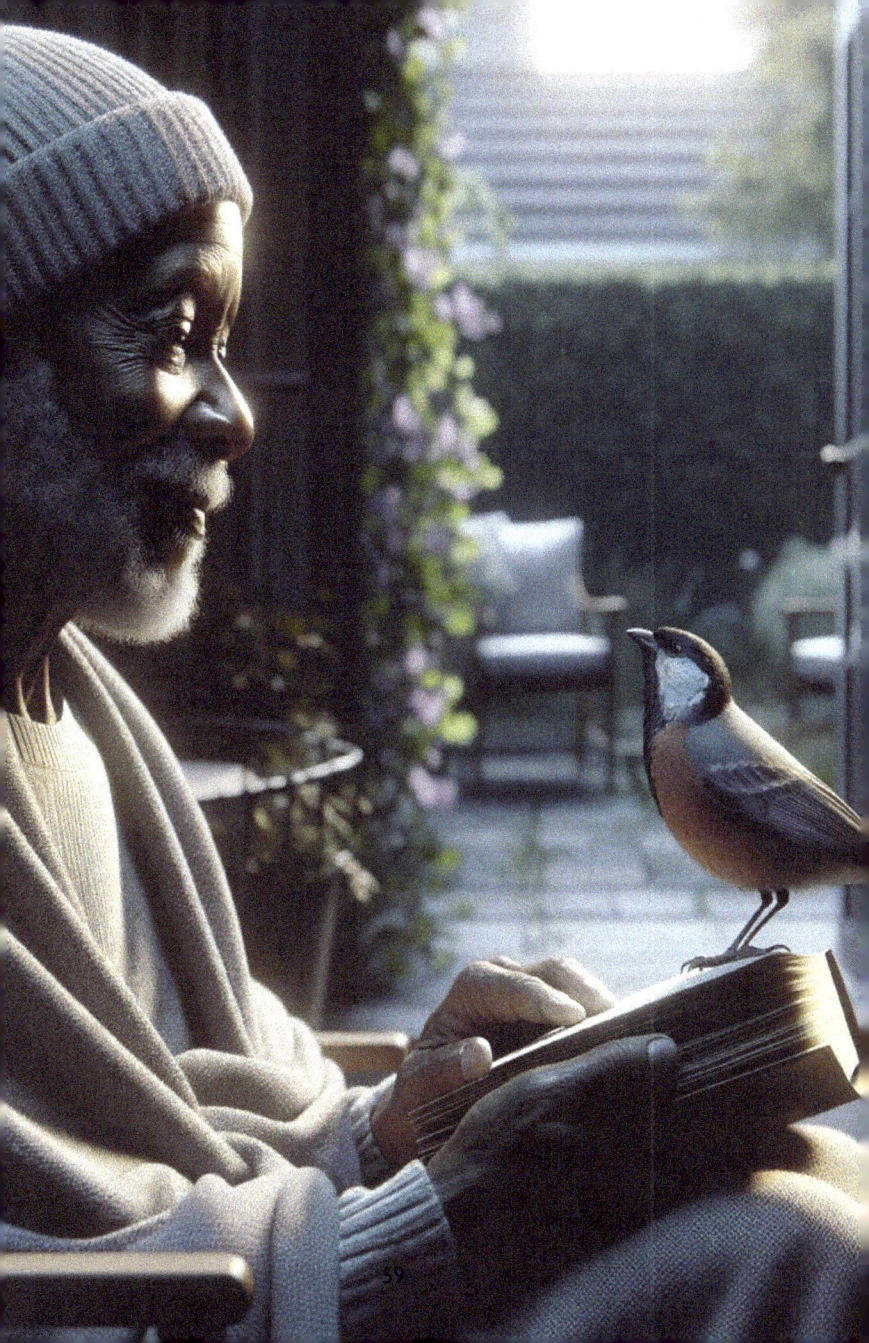

Activity:

Debrief & Doodle

Oh Love, I know this journey has been an eye opener. It is very likely that someone close to you has suffered from lack of access to good care. This hurt is a form of trauma. These experiences impact future experiences for you and those you love.

The environments around us and the components that make up these places have just about half the influence on our health. The places we live, our neighborhoods, schools, access to healthy foods, access to health care and opportunities for employment are the components of "social determinants of health." Social determinants of health contribute to about 50-60% of health outcomes (Lawry). The genes that are the building blocks of our bodies contribute about 30% of our health outcomes (Lawry).

If we looked at a map of the United States, we

would see trends in longevity of life based on where people live and what is available in their zip code (e.g., opportunities for employment, education, safety, healthy foods) (Minor, Artiga). We'd notice that people in Minnesota tend to live to an average age of just over 70 years old, and folks in West Virgina live to almost 64 years old (Brueck). Trying to understand data of a whole state is large and hard. So, I'll try to make it more realistic.

When we drill down further, it is obvious that residents of the most marginalized communities (e.g., socially vulnerable) have a much shorter length of life. Washington D.C. neighborhoods demonstrate this on a touchable scale. One D.C. community group (White people) is outliving another D.C. community group (Black people) by 32.9 years. The 10 miles between these D.C. communities equates to a generation of people gone too soon and potential innovation lost. This pattern continues throughout multiple regions of the United States (CDC: ANV).

Do not despair, Love. Collectively, we can change these outcomes. The first step is recognizing what is at play. Then, make a strategy to LIVE better.

Color in Activity

Deep Breath In ...

EXHALE

It's OK to let it out. You are not alone in this battle. Intense stress keeps our bodies in fight or flight mode. Deep breathing helps the mind and body come back into balance under times of stress (Russo, Macmillan).

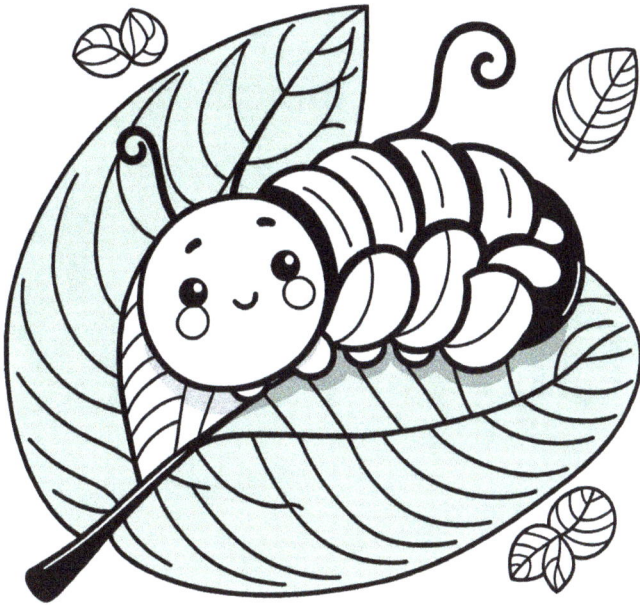

Just when the caterpillar
thought the world was over,
it became a

BUTTERFLY

—Chuang Tzu

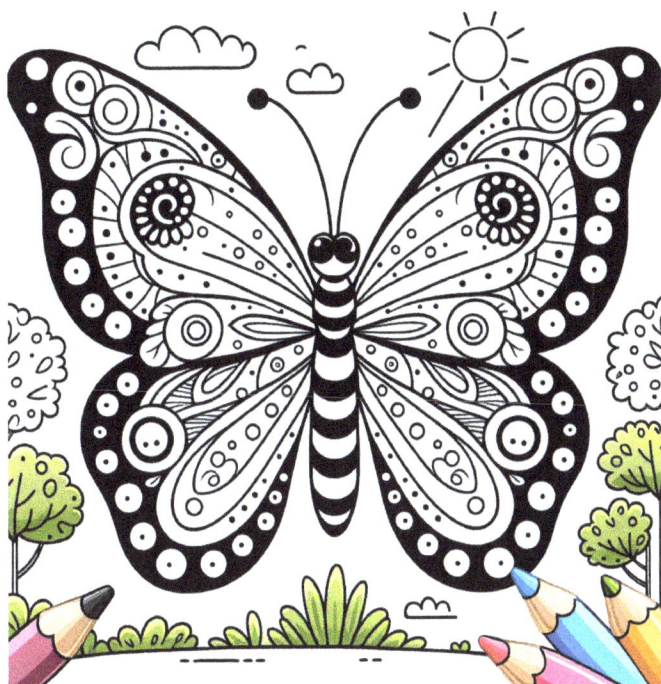

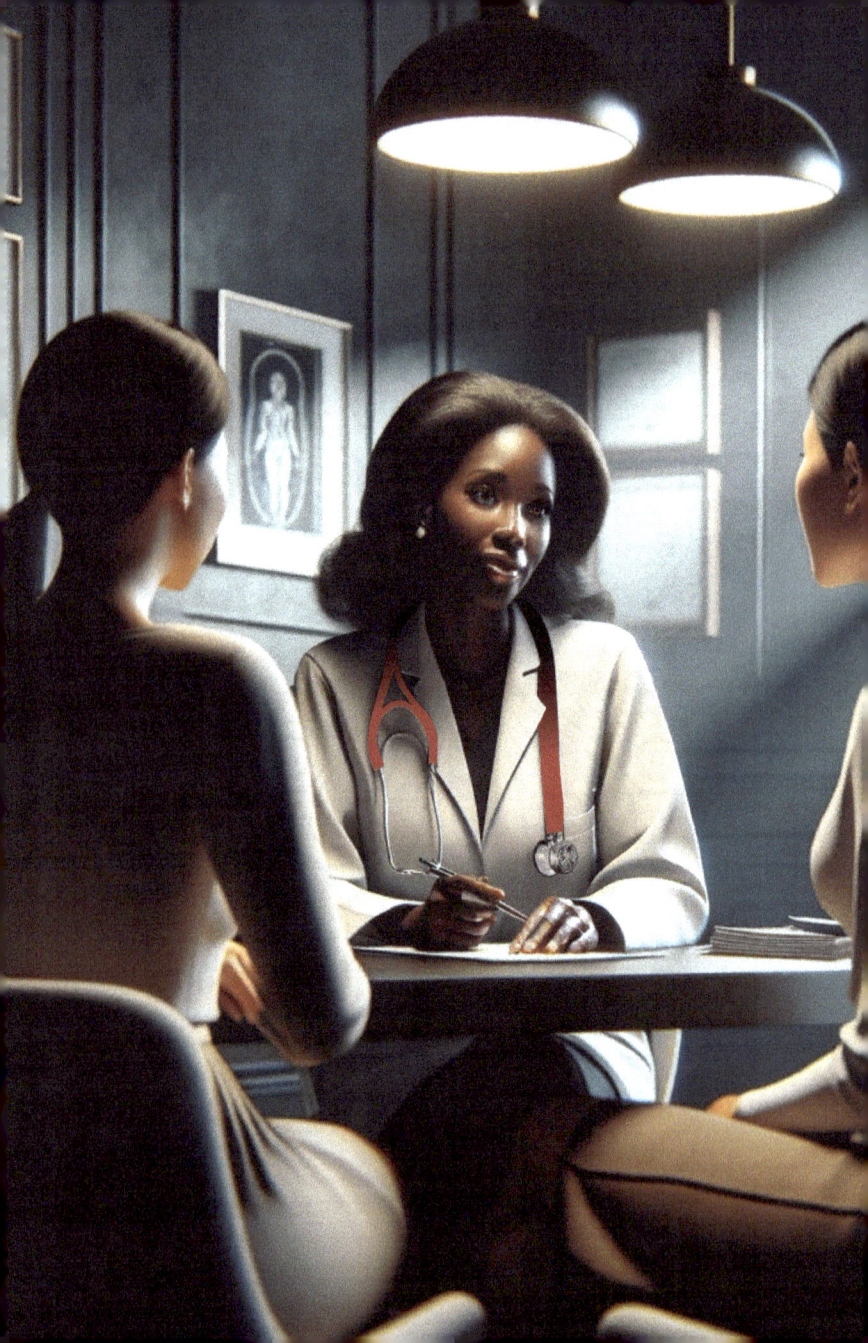

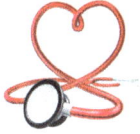

Chapter 4

LGBTQ+ Hope in Healthcare? Nope!

Compassionate Letter

It is a pleasure to meet you. Oh my heart, you made me wonder: Why are you so cold? Then I thought about it, and I understood. You can't tell from looking at me that I have nothing but compassion for you. I know other providers have come across with judgement in their eyes and actions. My only hope is that each human being can live their life from a place of comfort within their own skin. I'll try to clean it up a bit. Can I get a do-over? I'm so glad you made it into the office today. My name is Dr. Long. I go by she/her. I hope today is more of a conversation and the start of a partnership. What have your prior medical visits been like, and what do you hope to get from today's visit?

I am thankful that your new job encourages that you get a health physical, as it has been 15 years since you've seen a doctor or healthcare provider. I probably would not have gone back to the health center either after being treated that way. Can you tell me a bit about how you spend your days? I understand the road has been long. Someone felt uncomfortable at your last job, and it led to a roller coaster of pain. How did you survive the gap between jobs? Yes, your partner. I am thankful for her, as well.

Do the two of you have children? No, you hope to one day. Well, what is your plan for making that a reality? Have you thought of who will carry the pregnancy? Yes, you. That makes this visit even more exciting. Let's check your health to give you the best shot to support a healthy pregnancy. Can we do screening tests to check your heart, kidneys, thyroid, uterus? I suggest that everyone get checked for common infections. May I check you for possible infections, as well? I also have a few questions to screen your mood and mental health.

No, I'm sorry to offend. I just want you, your partner and the family you create to be healthy. I believe that taking a holistic approach to healthcare allows us to live our fullest lives.

Now, I can see the ice melting from your heart. Your eyes sparkled with hope that a new and better chapter has begun. You think there just might be hope in healthcare.

Down to Earth explanation

LGBTQ+ Preventative Health Observations. Many barriers exist that reduce the opportunities for LGBTQ+ patients to get routine medical care. Many people who identify as LGBTQ+ often forgo preventative health screenings, which allows treatable conditions to move to the realm of untreatable (Stanford). Access to respectful and supportive routine healthcare can extend the length and quality of LGBTQ+ lives (Maybank, Boyle) and increase the chances of patients returning for follow-up care (Deutsch).

Gender-affirming health centers for people who identify as LGBTQ+ are places that extend culturally appropriate care (Howard Brown Health) from a place of humility and respect for each person that presents for care (Deutsch). These centers are intent on reducing intentional and unintentional trauma often experienced in typical health facilities. Gender-affirming health centers are intentional in creating a hospitable space where providers are trained in and practice "cultural humility" (honoring the humanity and dignity of each person they care for) (Howard Brown). Inclusion is visible at the affirming health center through: opportunities for patient "self-designation of gender identity" from the first point of contact; explicit, publicly viewable LGBTQ+ Patient Standards of Care (Howard Brown); gender neutral restrooms; pronoun identification on staff badges; publicly available staff training materials that center inclusion; and offering comprehensive care that focuses on physical and socioemotional wellness of the people served. Local health centers may implement the previously mentioned gender-affirming strategies as a starting place to build its unique culture that centers respect for all people. Patient engagement for health center design would be ideal. Patients have invaluable insight to guide clinicians in their care as experts of their own bodies and lived experiences (Long).

Care Considerations

Innate gender expression needs no cure or conversion. Each person should be able to live their most authentic life in safety and wellness.

Healthcare services should be tailored to the unique person that presents for care. This will allow people to live their best lives.

U.S. Quick Facts

LGBTQ+
Health

Discrimination & Disrespect
in Healthcare Settings

• An unimaginably high number of LGBTQ+ people avoid seeking care (Deutsch) due to prior disrespect and discrimination by healthcare providers.

• It is common for people to avoid or delay medical care when sick or injured for fear of being disrespected or mistreated because of their gender identity (Fenway Health).

• Care at Gender-Affirming health centers for LGBTQ+ people can extend the quality and span, while increasing the chances of return for, healthcare (Maybank, Deutsch).

LGBTQ+ Resources Gender-Affirming Healthcare Center Finder/Locator: Planned Parenthood link https://www.plannedparenthood.org/learn/gender-identity or call 1-800-230-7526.

TransHealthCare gender-affirming surgical care link https://www.transhealthcare.org/find-surgeon/

Resources for Parents/Supporters of LGBTQ+ Loved Ones:

• Planned Parenthood link https://www.plannedparenthood.org/learn/parents/identity or call 1-800-230-7526.

• What is Gender-Affirming Care? link https://www.aamc.org/news-insights/what-gender-affirming-care-your-questions-answered (AAMC).

LGBTQ+ Youth

• LGBTQ+ Youth are at greater risk for physical and socioemotional health conditions (Hafeez).

• Physical health matters to be aware of: tobacco, drug and alcohol use (healthypeople.gov), sexually transmitted diseases, cardiovascular disease and obesity (Hafeez).

• Socioemotional health matters to be aware of: "bullying, isolation, rejection, anxiety, depression, and suicide" (Hafeez).

• Attempted suicide at rates 2-3 times higher among LGBTQ+ youth (Healthypeople.gov, Restar).

• A lack of stable housing is disastrous for LGBTQ+ Youth (Stanford, 19, 20, 21 healthypeople.gov).

• Almost "40% of all young people experiencing homelessness" are LGBTQ+ (Hafeez).

Resources:

• **Suicide and Crisis Lifeline** Call or SMS (text) **988** for help 24 hours a day. Multiple languages. Se habla Español. Llame **988**.

• Alcohol, Opioid, Drug Use Assistance **SAMHSA's National Helpline**, 1-800-662-HELP (4357) or TTY: 1-800-487-4889. Text your zip code to 435748 (HELP4U) all day everyday in multiple languages.

• **MarleyAyo's EnterWell** program helps companies, organizations, institutions to co-create strategies to center joy and build healthy inclusive communities. Email: connect@marleyayo.com

• **Planned Parenthood link** https://www.plannedparenthood.org/learn/gender-identity or call 1-800-230-7526.

Housing Resources:

• **The Trevor Project** or https://www.thetrevorproject.org/

• **Call The 1-800-RUNAWAY** (1-800-786-2929) "mission of the National Runaway Safeline (NRS) is to keep America's runaway, homeless and at-risk youth safe and off the streets."

• Call or text **988** "If you or someone you know is struggling or in crisis" (SAMSHA). Se habla Español, Llame 988.

• Rape Abuse & Incest National Network (RAINN) Hotline 1-800-656-HOPE (4673) anytime day or night

LGBTQ+ Elders

• LGBTQ+ elders are 2 times more "likely to be single and live alone" (SAGE Get Involved).

• When critical or life-threatening illnesses occur, familial supports may not exist as they may for non-LGBTQ+ people (NHCPO). This can be a challenge with healthcare choices or end-of-life decision-making when LGBTQ+ elders are unable to speak for themselves.

• LGBTQ+ elders experience significant challenges to high quality healthcare services due to an absence of culturally competent providers, limited social services and isolation (Healthypeople.gov, Sharman).

• Call **877-360-LGBT "SAGE's National LGBT Elder Hotline** is available 24 hours a day, 7 days a week" to speak with you in English or Spanish for older adult support.

• **Create End-of-Life Documents** to have your wishes known, empower your family of choice, and reduce chances of imposed guardianship (Prachniak, SAGE, Sharman).

Routine Healthcare Prevention

• **Healthcare** for LGBTQ+ people is often deferred or not obtained secondary to prior traumatic experiences with healthcare providers (Stanford, Sharman).

• **Sexual and gender** minority (SGM) people experience impacts to the length and quality of their life from diseases that can be managed with early treatment.

• **Lesbians** are less likely to get preventive services for cancer (healthypeople.gov).

• **Gay men** are at higher risk of HIV and multiple sexually transmitted infections. Communities of color are the most significantly impacted (healthypeople.gov).

• **Transgender** people have a lower quality of life and poorer mental health without gender-affirming care (Restar).

• **Nonbinary/Gender Diverse** people experience lower safety and increased discrimination in the absence of gender affirming care (NLHEC).

HIV Prevention

• **Pre-Exposure Prophylaxis** (PrEP) is an evidence-based medication that can reduce the risk of getting infected by HIV.

• "**PrEP** reduces the risk of getting HIV from sex by about 99% when taken as prescribed" (CDC PrEP).

• **Find a clinic** or provider that prescribes PrEP at link https://locator.hiv.gov/

• **Ready, Set, PrEP** offers free HIV PrEP to those that qualify: https://readysetprep.hiv.gov/

• **Planned Parenthood PrEP Services and Resources** https://www.plannedparenthood.org/learn/stds-hiv-safer-sex/hiv-aids/prep or call 1-800-230-7526

RX FOR SELF-ADVOCACY

Questions to Ask for Gender-Affirming LGBTQ+ Healthcare:

• What routine health/preventative health screening is needed for me?

• What is the center's policy on gender-affirming health education for providers?

• How does the center offer discrete care and treatment? Are there options for remote access?

• What mental health services are offered here?

• What gender-affirming therapies are available here?

• Do you offer services like PrEP to reduce the chances of infection?

• Do you offer substance use services for drugs and alcohol?

• Do you have resources for safe housing?

• "I want you to know" cards by George Washington School of Medicine & Health Sciences provides additional tools for guiding your conversation with your provider. Cards are available in English, Spanish and Chinese at https://cancercontroltap.smhs.gwu.edu/news/i-want-you-know.

Didn't I See That in the News?

Late breaking research reported that 47% of LGBTQ+ people have experienced feeling invalidated or dismissed by a "doctor, nurse, technician, or therapist" within the last two years (Mastroianni) 15% of LGBTQ+ people surveyed reported that providers told them "their symptoms were 'all in their head'" (Mastroianni). Such discounting, disrespectful power play is known as gaslighting. Of note, similar gaslighting experiences have been reported by people who are advanced in age and other marginalization communities (e.g., women and people of color) when they seek medical care.

In addition to not being heard by their doctors, 18% of LGBTQ+ people have experienced trauma at the hands of their medical providers, and 10% said they have experienced "some form of medical discrimination" (Mastroianni). These terrible experiences are often reasons LBGTQ+ community members put off seeking medical care until the situation is dire. Each time a person experiences such trauma and gaslighting from medical providers, it decreases the patient's overall health and increases mental distress from PTSD, anxiety and depression.

The entire medical community is not all the same. There are gender-affirming centers and providers out there. LGBTQ+ people, you are seen. You are seen. And you are worthy to be seen as your entire wonderful self. In this partnership for great health and a full life, I'll let you say what you need for yourself. To see and hear LGBTQ+ voices on seeking healthcare, open the following link: https://www.lgbtqiahealtheducation.org/video/lgbt-voices-perspectives-on-healthcare/.

Together
we can navigate
a safe and healthy
way forward.

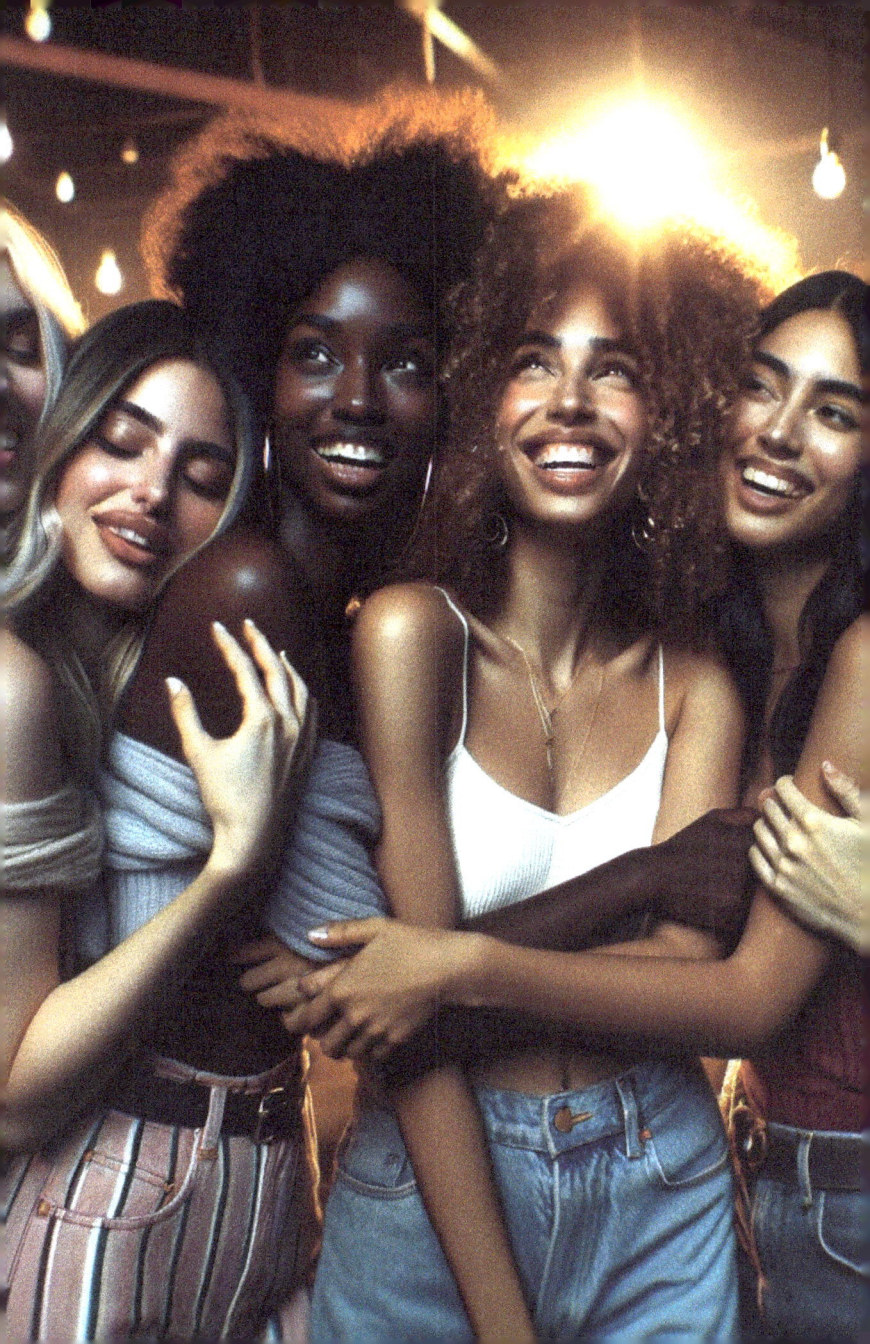

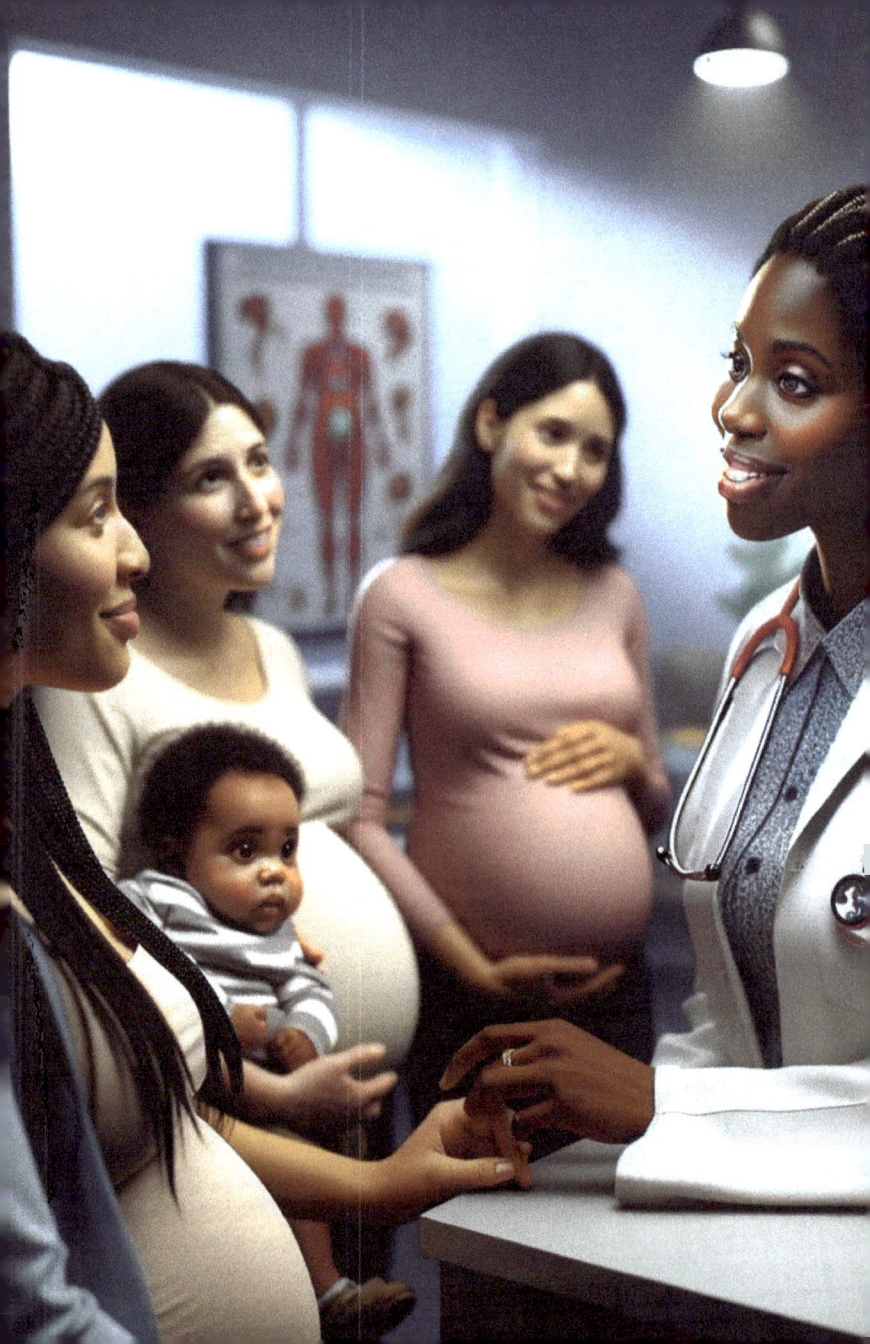

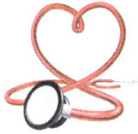

Chapter 5

Pregnancy Pains & Precautions

MATERNAL & INFANT HEALTH
Compassionate Letter

Double Loves, you've made it to the second half of your pregnancy! Yes, I understand the nausea has been a mess. Your weight is on the lower side. What have you been able to eat? Do you have access to healthy foods? Yes, you do. However, you find it hard to eat with your partner.

They have been so stressed out over the baby, expenses and the dread of no protected time to spend with you and baby after delivery. I can see you are stressed out for them. My dear, it's so important that you get a handle on this. Excessive stress shows up as physical manifestations in your body. Technically, this is allostatic overload (Guidi, Geronimus, McEwen). Your body's response to stressors – be them physical, psychological, social, or emotional – puts baby at risk of being born early or born small (from reduced nutrient flow to baby) and increases your personal risk of seizures/toxemia (Coussons-Read). I've seen these stressors show up in the body as elevated blood pressure, trouble sleeping, upset stomach, vomiting and more.

Do you have anyone nearby that you can lean on for support? No one, uhm. Would you consider meeting a group of moms-to-be that are at a similar place in pregnancy? You might find support in this community. If you like, I can connect you to a perinatal therapy specialist for some customized one-on-one care and support. Yes, you've made my day. I'll arrange these resources right away.

How about your honey? Do they have a support system outside of you? This can be a really stressful time for the unpregnant parent. Many feel that things are out of control, and they are living through a scary movie. Families that have high pregnancy support and positive relationships at the time of birth have babies that do better. There is an increased chance that the babies will live to the age of 1 year old. These infants have a lower infant mortality (Alio) compared to families without support. Moms with high support have some wins, as well. These moms have lower risks of depression, smoking, and anxiety (Cheng). We have partnerships with organizations that support nonpregnant parents during pregnancy. Please take this flyer for one such group.

I know that pregnancy and the thoughts of raising a child in these times is stressful. Know that you have people cheering for you and your family. Know that for 200,000 years humans have been giving birth (Brittanica). Know that your team of caregivers are smart and competent. We will do everything possible for you and baby to have a healthy pregnancy and delivery.

Down to Earth explanation
Maternal/Obstetric Health Observations.

Pregnancy and delivery are very complex physical processes with many opportunities for things to go wrong along the way. Mom's physical and emotional safety are of great concern during pregnancy. Homicide by a person known to the expectant mother is the number one cause of peripartum (period of time around delivery including the 42 days after delivery (CDC) death for women in the United States (Harvard, BMJ). Being murdered around the time of pregnancy or delivery is more likely than having a pregnancy related medical condition and dying in the U.S. (Harvard). Uncontrolled high blood pressure and disease of heart muscle (or cardiomyopathy) are the leading causes of significant illness and health burden during and right after the time of pregnancy (Wallace, Coussons). "For every pregnancy-related death, there are" 10 times as many unexpected severe events during labor and delivery that result in real harm to the pregnant person's health (ACOG Elim).

Care Considerations

Not being alone and having a supportive community during and immediately after pregnancy have tremendously positive impact on moms (Cheng), babies (Tannis, Byerley, Cunningham) and partners (Anderson Small, ACOG GPC, Cheng). There are models to group pregnant people at similar stages (or cohort) in prenatal care with individual tailored support as needed for the complexity of each pregnancy (ACOG GPC). Research reveals that cohort patients are more knowledgeable about the process of pregnancy, feel more empowered "for labor and delivery," report greater satisfaction with obstetrical care, and start breastfeeding more compared to people that had individual only prenatal care. There is no evidence to suggest "that group prenatal care causes harm" (ACOG GPC). Some organizations are even more forward thinking by shifting towards

Family-Oriented Care, "where the family as a whole is taken into account" (Anderson, Small).

"It takes a village to raise a child."— African Proverb

U.S. Quick Facts

Maternal/Obstetric Health Observation

Getting Killed During or Right After Pregnancy is a Public Health Crisis!

• Murder, more than pregnancy medical causes, is more likely to be the cause of death for pregnant and recently pregnant women (Harvard, Wallace).

• U.S. leads the world among high-income countries in gun deaths among pregnant women (ACOG Gun V, Everytown, Wallace).

• Just about 66% of perinatal attacks occurred in the home. The majority of fatal injuries were caused by a firearm (ex., handguns, rifles). Assault from sharp objects then strangulation (or getting choked out) were second and third most commonly used tactics (Wallace).

• Black women face substantially higher risk of being killed around the time of pregnancy than White or Latinx women (Harvard).

Pearls for Further Explanation

• **Call 1.800.799.SAFE** (7233) or text "START" to 88788. TTY for the hearing-impaired at (800) 787-3224 anytime day or night to get help from the National Domestic Violence Hotline.

• **Rape Abuse & Incest National Network** (RAINN) Hotline 1-800-656-HOPE (4673) anytime day or night.

Support resources for families of gun violence during pregnancy:

• National Domestic Violence Hotline https://www.thehotline.org/

• **Everytown** https://everytownsupportfund.org/everytown-survivor-network/resources-for-victims-and-survivors-of-gun-violence/

Medical Pregnancy

Medical Pregnancy Complications

• The health and wellbeing of a pregnant person has a direct impact on the health on the child born.

• Black women have the highest pregnancy related death rate at 41.4% (AHA Maternity).

• Indigenous women have a pregnancy-related death rate of 26.5%.

• The U.S. average pregnancy-related death rate is 17.3% (AHA Maternity).

Find Free or Reduced Cost Prenatal Care:

• U.S. Health & Human Services Call 1-800-311-BABY (1-800-311-2229) - This toll-free telephone number will connect you to the Health Department in your area code.

• Para informacion en Español, llame 1-800-504-7081

• Free Personal Nurse
https://www.nursefamilypartnership.org/first-time-moms/

Resources for Partners

• **CHOP (Children's Hospital of Philadelphia)** https://www.chop.edu/centers-programs/center-fetal-diagnosis-and-treatment/online-support-groups-new-and-expecting-parents

• **Babylist for New Dads** https://www.babylist.com/hello-baby/help-new-parents

• **First-Time Dads & Partners** https://www.nursefamilypartnership.org/first-time-moms/expectant-fathers/

• **LBGTQ+** https://lgbtmummies.com/our-support-groups

• **P³ (Pregnancy and Parenting Partners)** https://www.pregnancyandparentingpartners.org/p3-participants

• **CDC Hear Her™ Campaign** https://www.cdc.gov/hearher/index.html

Infant Complications From Pregnancy

Medical Pregnancy Complications

• The U.S. Infant Mortality rate of 5.42 deaths per 1,000 live births (Faststats) is the highest amongst high-income countries in the world (Petrullo).

• "Low birth weight and prematurity, which occur in 8% and 11.4% of all US births, are leading causes of immediate and chronic health problems for children" (Cheng).

• "NEARLY 50% of all infant deaths" in U.S. were linked to "pregnancy complications, low birth weight, and prematurity" (Cheng).

• Group prenatal care (or cohort pregnancy care) is linked to improved birth outcomes for infants. There are significantly fewer preterm births and NICU (neonatal intensive unit) stays, improved birth weights for infants, higher levels of breastfeeding, and increased patient/provider satisfaction with cohort care (ACOG GPC).

• Black women had a significant reduction in preterm births with group prenatal care (Cheng).

• "There is no evidence that suggests that group prenatal care causes harm" (Cheng).

• Some organizations are using "pediatric group care models" to bolster care (Cheng).

Resources:

National Resources for Families per Nurse-Family Partnership https://www.nursefamilypartnership.org/national-resources-for-moms/

Maternal Complications from Pregnancy

• Massive bleeding after delivery (or post-partum hemorrhage), cardiovascular disease, and self-inflicted harm are leading complications to U.S. pregnancies.

• Women in rural communities die at rates significantly higher than women in more urban communities from pregnancy complications (PMSS).

• Women age 40+ are at almost 8 times the risk of death from pregnancy than women under 25 years old (Hoyert).

• Group prenatal care (or cohort pregnancy care) has been linked to significantly fewer preterm births and NICU (neonatal care unit) stays, higher levels of breastfeeding, and increased patient/provider satisfaction with cohort care (ACOG GPC).

• Patients comment on being better prepared for labor and delivery and have greater prenatal knowledge from participating in group prenatal care (Cheng).

• Black women had the greatest impact to preterm birth by participating in group prenatal care according to the largest high quality research study on the matter (ACOG GPC).

Post-Partum Hemorrhage

Massive bleeding from damaged blood vessels is a major cause of death after pregnancy (Wallace, PMSS, ACOG 11). There are evidence-based practices to improve response and treatment to unexpected events.

• **Safe Motherhood Bundles** (ACOG 11)
   - Readiness (every patient)
   - Recognition (every unit)
   - Response (every time)
   - Reporting (every unit learning)

Cardiovascular Disease
(Hypertension, Cardiomyopathy)

Leading causes of deaths during pregnancy are cardiovascular in nature:

• Elevated blood pressure and heart muscle weakness are leading causes of death during pregnancy (Wallace, PMSS, ACOG II).

• Cardiomyopathy (weakness of heart muscle)

• Indigenous women have the highest rates of death (14.5%) from cardiomyopathy around the times of pregnancy and delivery (AHA Maternity).

High Blood Pressure Resources:

• ACOG FAQs: Preeclampsia and High Blood Pressure During Pregnancy https://www.acog.org/womens- health/faqs/preeclampsia-and-high-blood-pressure-during-pregnancy)

• Preeclampsia Foundation https://www.pre-eclamp-sia.org/public/signs-and symptoms.

Heart Function Resources:

• Cardiomyopathy https://www.heart.org/en/health-topics/cardiomyopathy/what-is- cardiomyopathy-in-adults/peripartum- cardiomyopathy-ppcm

Suicide

• Suicide is a leading cause of death in the U.S. for people that are pregnant or recently pregnant (Katella).

• Depression after pregnancy, postpartum depression, increases the risk of suicide (Katella).

• Having conditions such as anxiety, bipolar disorder and substance use disorder were linked to increased suicide risk (Akkas).

Suicide and Crisis Lifeline

Call or SMS (text) 988 for help 24 hours a day. Se habla Español, Llame 988.

Depression

ACOG FAQs: Depression During Pregnancy (https://www.acog.org/womens- health/faqs/depression-during-pregnancy)

Partner Abuse and Violence

National Domestic Violence Hotline Call 1.800.799. SAFE (7233) or text "START" to 88788

Resources for Partners

• Healthy nonpregnant partners (e.g., lovers, spouses, intimate friends) can have a positive impact on the pregnant partner's health and possibly the health of the baby (Cheng, Alio).

• **CHOP (Children's Hospital of Philadelphia)** https://www.chop.edu/centers-programs/center-fetal-diagnosis-and-treatment/online-support-groups-new-and-expecting-parents

• **Babylist for New DADs**
https://www.babylist.com/hello-baby/help-new-parents

• **First-Time Dads and Partners**
https://www.nursefamilypartnership.org/first-time-moms/expectant-fathers/

• **LBGTQ+**
https://lgbtmummies.com/our-support-groups

• **P³ (Pregnancy and Parenting Partners)**
https://www.pregnancyandparentingpartners.org/p3-participants

• **CDC Hear Her™ Campaign**
https://www.cdc.gov/hearher/index.html

• **Free Personal Nurse**
https://www.nursefamilypartnership.org/first-time-moms/

RX FOR SELF-ADVOCACY

Questions to ask about Maternal/Obstetric Health (Pregnancy Pains & Precautions):

• What is my blood pressure? **Ask this question at every doctor/healthcare provider visit after the second half of your pregnancy until 3 months after delivery.**

• What is my blood type?

• What are the signs of hemorrhage that I should look out for? How long should I look for hemorrhage signs (how many weeks after delivery am I at risk for postpartum hemorrhage)?

• Does your hospital use the "Safe Motherhood Bundles" to care for pregnant women?

• CDC Conversation Starter for Pregnant and Postpartum Women provides additional tools for guiding your conversation with your provider. The script and downloads are available from the following link: https://www.cdc.gov/hearher/pregnant-postpartum-women/index.html .

Didn't I See That in the News?

From the Olympics to near death, then back to the Olympics is the lived truth for the 11-time Olympic medal winning Track & Field Star Allyson Felix. Her health care team picked up that something was not right at a routine prenatal visit two months before her due date.

That day, Allyson went from having a joy filled routine pregnancy visit to an immediate anxiety producing admission into the hospital. Her blood pressure was too high, and she was showing other signs of pre-eclampsia, the percussor to toxemia. Her doctor was concerned that Allyson or her unborn baby could suffer life-threatening complications, if treatment was not provided quickly.

Ultimately, medication alone was not enough to control Allyson's pre-eclampsia. She was rushed for an emergency C-section surgery to deliver her first child at 32 weeks of pregnancy. That was 5 weeks earlier than the baby would be considered full-term and 8 weeks less than the ideal 40-week pregnancy delivery.

Fortunately, Allyson and her pre-term baby survived the ordeal. Her family gets to enjoy the both of them in great health. The world got to give Allyson a standing ovation at her 11th Olympic medal win after the birth of her daughter.

To hear Allyson share her story personally, click the link that follows. There are other brave women who have shared their stories, as well. https://www.cdc.gov/hear-her/personal-stories/index.html

CDC Hear Her™ Campaign:

"Unexpected Pregnancy Complications: Allyson Felix's Story"

Hoping for the day that we can archive such stories because healthcare will advance in the U.S. for moms, babies and families.

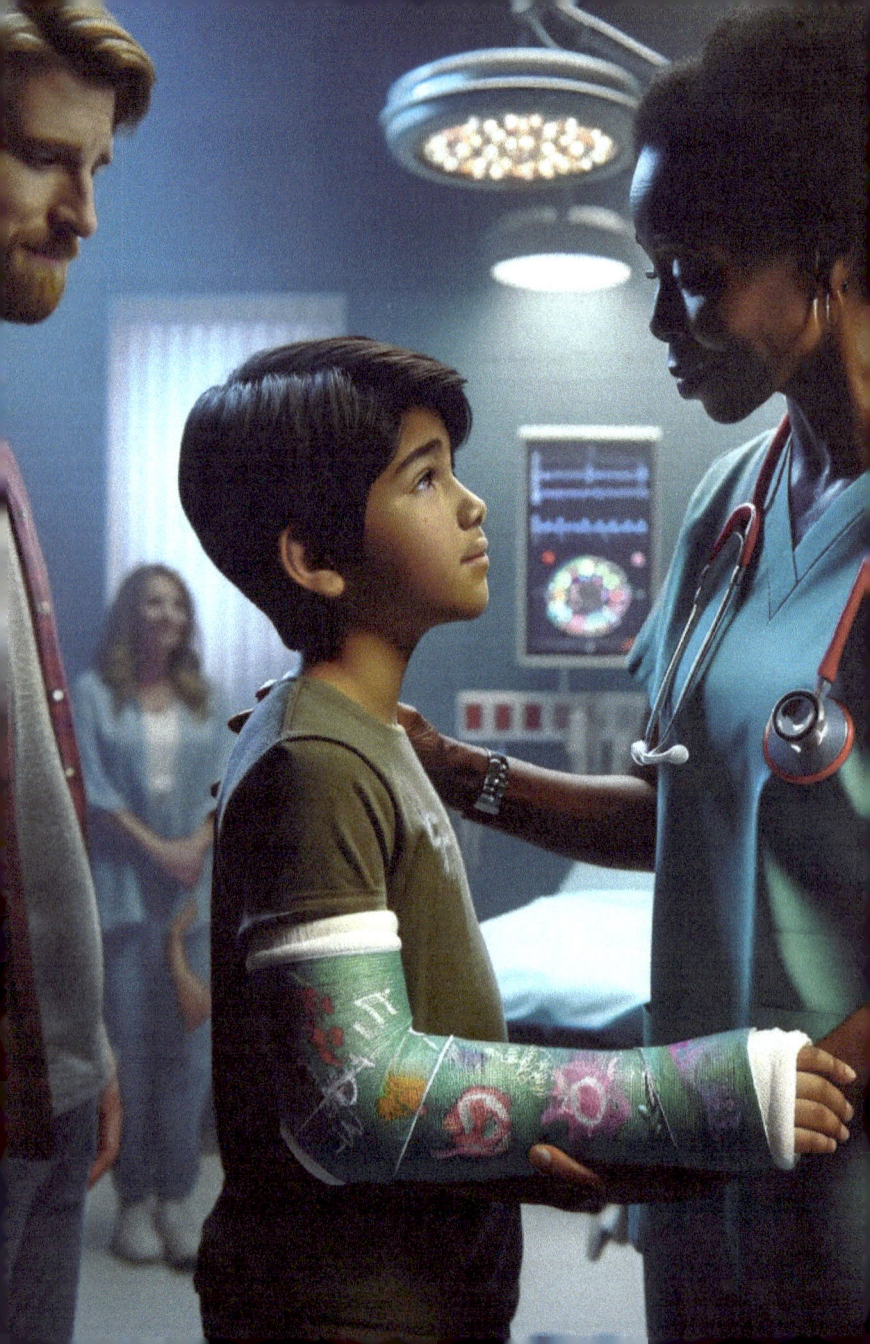

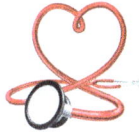

Chapter 6

Tiny Hurts.
No, Children
Feel Trauma, Too

(PEDIATRIC ACCIDENTS & INJURIES)

Compassionate Letter

Tiny love, I know you are scared. You had no idea that a trip to the playground would end this way. Yes, your ouwie hurts. I understand. How about a little ice and medicine for the pain as a start?

You're still scared? The ambulance ride was really loud! Your parents are right here. Want to cuddle with them? What about a new stuffy animal friend to cuddle on, too?

Parents, are you breathing? I think your heart rates are faster than mine. Take a breath. Your tiny love took a big fall and hurt their arm. I could only imagine the alarm you felt when the school called. The EMS Team is a great crew. They knew just what to do. Now, here in the Emergency Department (ED), we will keep the good energy going.

We will do x-rays next, to figure out what's going on. Tiny love, a ginormous camera machine will take a special picture of your arm. As soon as it is done, we can all look at the images together. Oh yes, it is broken. We know just what to do. We will give you some silly medicine, right by your nose. Then we will help put the bones back into their regular spot. We'll finish off with a cool splint or cast. Would you like to pick a special color? You'll have a big story to tell and something to share when you go back to school. Then you and your friends can put art on your cast to make it just your own. Would you like us to make a splint for your stuffy, too?

Parents, how are you? Will you be okay? What do you need? Tiny love is very brave. They have done better than many adult patients with the same injury. Your sweet child will have this cast for a few weeks, then will be back to their old selves. I am so thankful it was just the arm that got broken.

I know this whole thing has been scary for everyone. Would you all like to have our Trauma Specialist come in and chat for a bit about how to get through this? Wonderful, I'll ask that they stop by right away.

Down to Earth explanation

Accidents and the resulting trauma are the #1 cause of death for people aged 1-19 years old in the United States. Many more youth experience non-life-threatening injuries each year. Many times the non-life-threatening injuries can do just as much emotional and mental damage as a more severe injury (CDC TIC). Guns (and other firearms), cars, bikes, and pools are among the many sources of injury to children. A large portion of these injuries could be prevented, if safer practices on equipment and protective gear were utilized (Hassanein). Nineteen percent of children have PTSD (post-traumatic stress disorder) after sustaining an injury (SAMHSA T). Children lose a significant number of days of education in school because of injuries. Less obvious, parents and caregivers lose days of work and of potential income while caring for injured children. The ripples of childhood trauma are notable beyond the family unit and extend into the community (Hassanein).

Long-term, unaddressed trauma can reduce the life span and increase the chance of illness as the children become adults. "Toxic stress from Adverse Childhood Experiences (ACEs) can negatively affect children's brain development, immune systems, and stress-response systems. These changes can affect children's attention, decision-making, and learning" (CDC ACEs, Bhushan, Burke Harris). Overtime, diseases like hypertension, heart disease and cancer begin to show up from the toxic stress. High doses of adversity not only affect brain structure and function. They affect the developing immune system, developing hormonal systems and even the way the DNA in our genes work. "With the right intervention, you can prevent and even sometimes reverse these huge health problems" (Burke Harris/Raz).

Care Considerations

Immediate care for the injuries that compromise thinking, breathing and other organ function is paramount. After the initial stabilization of the physical wounds/injuries, attention must shift to the mental and social health impacts of trauma. Dr. Hargarten suggest a biopsychosocial approach to trauma care (Hargarten). Bandages, surgeries and medications alone are not enough to help youth recover from trauma.

Many children experience post-traumatic stress disorder from trauma (Hargarten) or an adverse childhood event. The best care comes from healthcare teams deep with talent of "psychologists, social workers, and case managers, emergency physicians, trauma surgeons," etc. Each player on the team is key in addressing the other components of the disease to reduce post-traumatic stress disorder risk, ensure adequate follow-up with trauma-informed care, and partner with the community to address the social aspects of this disease. An array of short-term (hospital-based intervention/interrupter programs) and long-term programs are key tools in changing the impact of trauma (Hargarten).

Once patient care moves beyond just the bed-side, our youth will have a chance to truly heal and be whole. The data shows that strength-ening family centered support early in a child's life reaps dividends of high-quality life for that child and society as an adult (Felitti). Empow-ering youth with helpful tools to cope with life's stressors and challenges is another way forward, once they become survivors of ACEs (Felitti, CDC).

Limiting long term toxic stress within the child's body can improve their health as a grown-up. Adult survivors of ACEs were significantly more likely to attempt suicide, noted to abuse alcohol and drugs, smoke, report poorer over-all health (Felitti, Burke Harris), repeat a grade in school or have a personal encounter with the criminal justice system (Burke Harris).

U.S. Quick Facts

Pediatric Health Observations

Impact of Adverse Childhood Experiences (ACEs)

• **20-year reduction in length of life for a young person depending on a large number of ACEs they experience (Burke Harris)**

• Adverse Childhood Experiences are traumatic living circumstances children grow up in that are influenced by:

   - psychological, physical, or sexual abuse
   - violence against mothers
   - living with household members who were substance abusers, mentally ill or suicidal, or ever imprisoned (Felitti).

• The higher a person's ACE score, the worse health outcomes they had (Burke Harris/Raz).

• Almost 67% of U.S. Adults have a childhood ACE (Swedo) and 1 in 6 adults report 4+ ACEs by age 18 (CDC ACEs).

• ACEs were greatest amongst Indigenous Adult females who were unable to work or unemployed (CDC ACEs).

Pearls for Further Explanation

• Children could reach their full potential if ACEs can be prevented.

• **Protective measures include:**
  - physical and emotional safety
  - stability in relationships for children and households
  - high-quality preschools with family engagement
  - support for healthy dating skills (CDC ACEs).

Understanding Child Trauma
by SAMHSA

https://www.samhsa.gov/child-trauma/understanding-child-trauma

Safety Tips for Home, Away and Play from Healthychildren.org/American Academy of Pediatrics

https://www.healthychildren.org/English/safety-prevention/Pages/default.aspx

Physical Trauma

• "In 2020, firearm-related injuries became" the **#1 cause of death in U.S. for people 1-19** years old (CDC FastStats, Goldstick) with no signs of changing in the near future (KFF CT).

• Motor vehicle accidents, overdoses, then cancer are the next leading causes of youth deaths (USA Facts).

• Males are "86% of all victims of firearm death and 87% of nonfatal firearm injuries" (CDC Violence Prevention).

• "In 2020 alone, at least 125 toddlers and **children age 5 and under shot themselves or someone else**" (Schaechter).

• Out of sight is not out of mind with gun (pistol) storage. Children are bright and curious. They figure out how to access firearms (CDC Violence Prevention).

Gun Safety:

BE SMART

Secure all guns in your homes and vehicles.

Model responsible behavior around guns.

Ask about unsecured guns in other homes.

Recognize the role of guns in suicide.

Tell your peers to Be SMART.

https://besmartforkids.org/

Resources:

BeSMARTforKids.org
For tips or to get involved,
text SMART to 644-33
Free gun lock and safety information:
Project ChildSafe Safety Kit

https://projectchildsafe.org/safety/get-a-safety-kit/
(Project Child Safe).

Childhood Cancer

• There have been huge advances in cancer survival for children since the 1970s.

• 85% of U.S. children with cancer now survive 5 years or more (ACS Key Stats).

• **"If your child does develop cancer, it's important to know that it's extremely unlikely there is anything you or your child could have done to prevent it" (ACS Childhood).**

• Treatment of childhood cancer includes combinations of chemo (chemotherapy), radiation, immunotherapy (ACS Treating) or gene therapy.

• **HOPE** is important to hold on to. "Try to find both little and big things to hope for. Focus on keeping that hope by sharing it with your child, family, friends, and your child's medical care team so that they can share their hopes with you (Terao).

• **FEAR** is common. "It is okay to be afraid" (Terao). "If you find yourself having financial difficulties, do not hesitate to ask your child's doctor or social worker for help. Your child's medical team may be able to find financial resources that can help" (Terao).

• **TALK** to your child and the care team about the cancer. For tips to talk to your child, the National Cancer Institute has very helpful tips, guides and videos. https://www.cancer.gov/about-cancer/coping/caregiver-support/parents

Support for Families

National Children's Cancer Society (NCCS) 314.241.1600 or toll-free 800.5FAMILY (800.532.6459)

When Your Child Has Cancer
(ACS) common questions
800.227.2345, https://www.cancer.org/cancer/survivors hip/children-with-cancer.html

Childhood Overdose & Poisoning

• **#3 Cause of death** of children.

• This category **increased** by 83.6% from 2019 to 2020 from narcotics/hallucinogens (pills and street drugs) (USAFacts) and unintentional household poisonings (Goldstick).

"Every race and ethnicity had an increase in overdose deaths in 2021" (USAFacts).

Call 988 for assistance if you have thoughts of hurting yourself.

Llame 988 ayuda si tiene pensamientos de hacerse daño.

RX FOR SELF-ADVOCACY

Questions to Ask About Childhood Trauma & Illness

- How is my child's pain being controlled?

- What is the best course of treatment for my child?

- How do we help our child with the fear of the accident when we go home?

- What are the long-term consequences of this injury?

- Where can I go as a caregiver when I need help taking care of this child?

Didn't I See That in the News?

21st Century Children

It was already hard being a kid in this fast-paced, tech heavy world. Then COVID came and staying away from people you didn't live with became the norm.

Many children are carrying a heavy load of stress and anxiety with them at baseline. Then, if they get injured or sick, these feelings can escalate (Fraga).

Children want to be seen and involved in things that affect them. This is even more important when things seem out of control and are painful. A large number of children already have fear and angst of visiting doctors and nurses (Child Mind). Many know the shot, poke and pain are coming during their visit. Their tears and fears are real and ignoring them or downplaying them could cause harm and make the situation worse (Fraga). Digital distractions can often help make things better if used with perameters.

The Surgeon General reported, "whale social media may offer some benefits, there are ample indicators that social media can also pose a risk of harm to the mental health and wellbeing of children and adolescents. Social media use by young people is nearly universal, with up to 95% of young people ages 13-17 reporting using a social media platform and more than a third saying they use social media "almost constantly." "Children are exposed to harmful content on social media, ranging from violent and sexual content, to bullying and harassment. And for too many children, social media use is compromising their sleep and valuable in-person time with family and friends" (Murthy).

Childhood and adolescence are critical times for brain growth and development in a young person's life (Murthy). We, parents/caregivers, focus on what foods children nourish their bodies with. Similar considerations should be taken for what young people nourish their brains with. Inspiring and affirming social media content can change the impact youth receive from the platform.

We've lost generations of progress for children, families and society since COVID came. "After the onset of the pandemic specifically, there were significant year-over-year increases in children's diagnosed behavioral or conduct problems, decreases in preventive medical care visits, increases in unmet health care needs, and increases in the proportion of young children whose parents quit, declined, or changed jobs because of childcare problems" (Leburn-Harris).

It is clear that the "invisible population," the children of people who are incarcerated, are experiencing ongoing trauma and challenges as they attempt to live through an active ACE (Starting Early). "If having an incarcerated parent was classified as a chronic health condition, it would be the second most prevalent chronic condition in the United States for children— just behind asthma" (Starting Early). "African-American children are 9 times more likely and Hispanic children are 3 times more likely than White children to have a parent in prison" (Starting Early).

Thus, **adults must be mindful of the seen and unseen wounds** that the young people of today carry with them.

The Foundation "Focuses on the earliest years, because early investment lasts a lifetime" (Barnett/ Burke Harris).

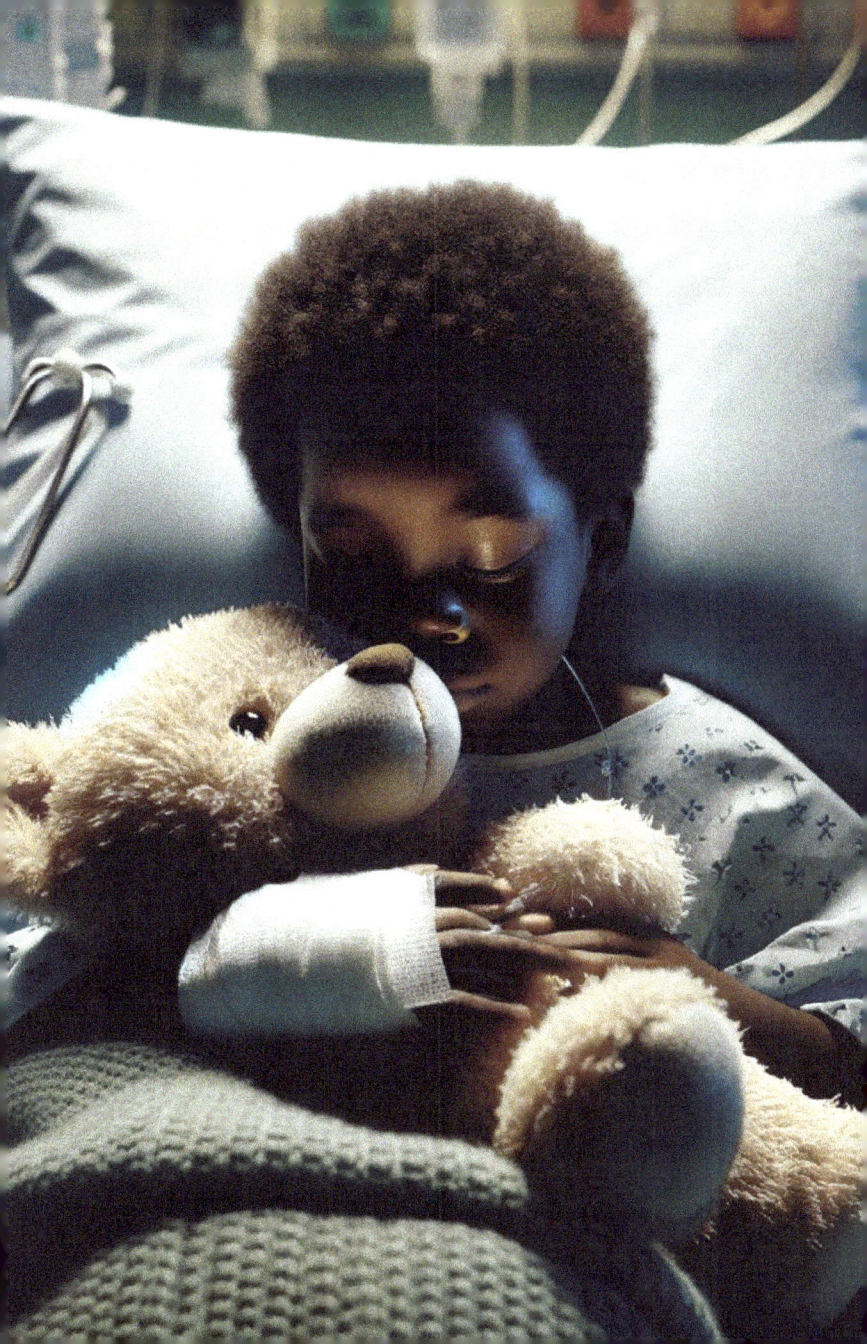

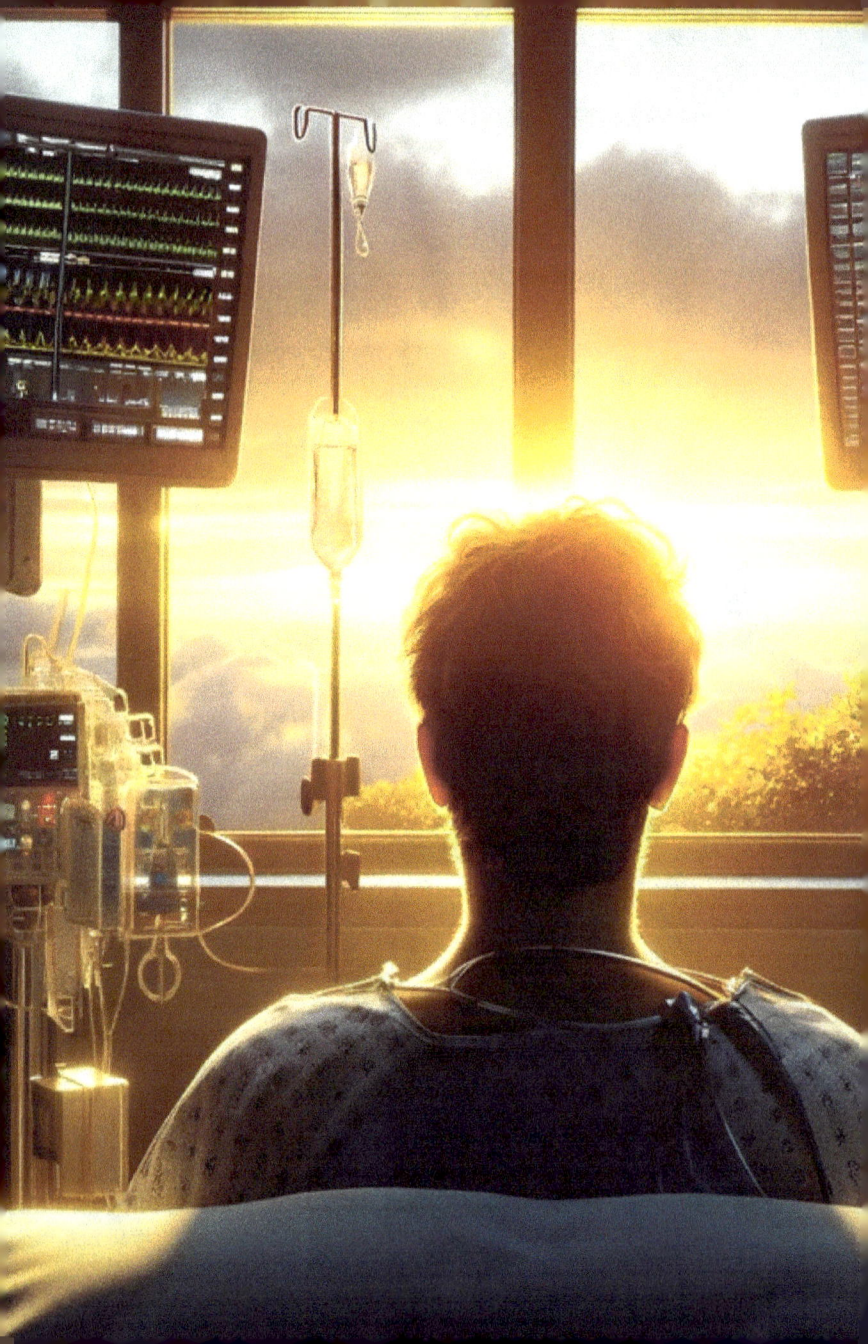

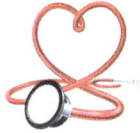

Chapter 7

Guns, Guns, Guns
(FIREARM TRAUMA)

Compassionate Letter

My dear, I hadn't planned on waking you in the middle of the night. Something terrible has happened tonight. Your son was shot multiple times and is in critical condition. No, no ma'am. I don't know the details. Only that a bystander called 9-1-1, and EMS got him here as soon as possible. Yes ma'am, he is alive. He has been critically injured. Are you able to come to the hospital safely?

I'm glad you were able to make it in so soon. Right now things are serious. He's in the best hands with our Trauma Surgeon. The road to recovery will be filled with trying times. We have a team of supporters to help your son and family with short- and long-term needs.

Is the rest of your family safe now? Oh ma'am, call your other children and let them know not to seek justice with their hands. We have law enforcement and community interrupters to help see that justice comes to pass. Right now, it is important to not do more harm in the streets. You know, "Peace is a lifestyle" (Ford), not one action. Would it be okay if one of our Trauma Counselors or Chaplain came and spent time with you? I will come back right away after I get an update from the team in the operating room.

The sun is now rising, and your son has made it safely to the recovery suite. The true road to recovery will be long. The physical wounds and holes will heal before the mental, emotional, and social wounds heal. Our teams are trained to interrupt the streets before more violence can pop off, support your son and your family in making safe moves after hospital discharge, and take the long journey with you all for holistic healing.

Any opportunity for a second chance at life and beating the odds is phenomenal. So many Black and Brown males are born into the world with an unstated terminal condition at birth. The condition is trauma and quite possibly death from firearms. There are two common outcomes and neither evokes hope. "Just lookin' at the facts. It's a coffin or a cell, if you young and you Black" (Hussle).

I absolutely understand why youth live for today. It's hard to really sit with such heavy facts. One dark side of this is that people can lose hope that they can shake such a predetermined fate. Collectively, survivors, the community, holistic healers, and elected officials can help change the odds and make it the new norm to live past 25 or 30-something years old!

> "Trauma feels so lonely."
> —Lauren London, Red Table Talk

Down to Earth explanation

Gun shot wounds are a type of firearm injury. Firearms contribute to 48,830 lives lost each year in the U.S. (Gramlich). These bullets do more than put a hole in physical tissue. They shatter communities more than bodies. On the individual level, bullets are small projectiles that directly injure the tissue they pierce and cause damage along the edge (perimeter) of the tract from their force, burning, soiling of carrier products (Shrestha) and broken bone fragments. Socially-emotionally, these projectiles destroy any sense of safety for the survivors of gun violence, their loves, and people who witnessed the event (Panchal).

Care Considerations

Immediate treatment involves caring for the critical physical threats to life and limb. Depending on the situation, sometimes just repair of the tissues damaged is needed. Other times, blood transfusions, broken bone repair and surgery are necessary. Depending on what part of the body was injured, healing times can vary. Skin may take 10 days or so to heal, if infection does not set in (Nagy). Infected wounds, nerve or internal organ injury may take several surgeries and months to a year to heal. The mental and emotional wounds may never heal.

Mentally, the trauma of the event can lock people into that day and rob them of hope and security in their bodies. Trauma-trained teams that focus on healing the entire person, not just the physical wounds, have better outcomes over traditional (physical wound) care alone. These teams of specialists are all trained to address every dimension of trauma: the physical, emotional, social and mental. They work in concert to make sure survivors and their families can be safe and thrive. Post-traumatic stress disorder (PTSD) is common after such a violent event. This may show up as reliving the event randomly or with triggers, nightmares, hallucinations, and keeping their guards up when out and about (Christensen).

It truly takes a comprehensive team that communicates and works well with survivors, their families and the local community to recover from firearm injury and gunshot trauma.

(Hargarten).

U.S. Quick Facts

Firearm Trauma Observations

Suicide

• Self-inflicted death makes up the #1 cause of firearm death.

• "Suicides have long accounted for the majority of U.S. gun deaths."

• "54% of all gun-related deaths in the U.S. were suicides (26,328), while 43% were murders (20,958)," in 2021 (Gramlich).

• **Males 75+** years old commit suicide the most (NIHM).

• Females age 45-64 are the most likely to complete the act of suicide for that sex.

• Suicide rates are 4 times higher for children who live in a home with a gun (Schaechter).

• Since the pandemic, there is a rise in suicide among young adults (Stobbe).

• Firearms are the #1 cause of death for children and teens in the U.S. (McGough).

• Homicide deaths happen way more often than suicide deaths between ages 15-19 year olds (Stobbe, McGough).

• A small portion of youth firearm injuries are unintentional (McGough). Greater than 33% happened in the "homes of their friends, neighbors, or relatives" (Schaechter).

• Recent "increases were seen in homicide rates for young Black and Hispanic people in the U.S." (Stobbe).

Pearls for Further Explanation

• **Call 988 for assistance if you have thoughts of hurting yourself.**

• **Para ayuda en Español, llame al 988.**

Gun Safety:

BE SMART

Secure all guns in your homes and vehicles.

Model responsible behavior around guns.

Ask about unsecured guns in other homes.

Recognize the role of guns in suicide.

Tell your peers to Be SMART.

https://besmartforkids.org/

Homicide
(Violence Against Others Resulting in Death)

• Homicide deaths happen way more than suicide deaths between ages 15-19 years old (Stobbe, McGough).

• A small portion of youth firearm injuries are unintentional (McGough). Greater than 33% happened in the "homes of their friends, neighbors, or relatives" (Schaechter).

• "Increases were seen in homicide rates for young Black and Hispanic people in the U.S." (Stobbe).

• Survivors of gun violence, young and old, have increased anxiety, depression, PTSD, and health conditions and substance use disorders (KFF CT, Burke/Raz, SAMSHA T).

• For the last 20 years, gun violence has been the **#1 cause of death for Black children and teens** (USA Facts).

RX FOR SELF-ADVOCACY

Questions to Ask About Firearm Trauma:

• What should I lookout for with my wounds and with healing?

• How will I ever be safe in this community again?

• How do violence Interrupters and police work together to catch the people that did this?

• Can you refer me to a Trauma-informed therapist?

**Ask friends and family that will have your children in their home how they store their guns. Think strongly about letting your children play in homes that do not store guns unloaded and unlocked.* *

"An abnormal reaction to an abnormal situation is normal behavior." —Victor Frankl, *Man's Search for Meaning*

Didn't I See That in the News?

Mrs. Mariah Clare

This just might workout. The kids seem to be adjusting to the divorce as best as one could expect. This time their visit with Dad went pretty smoothly. Of course, he could have a few more minutes to play with the kids. I know this is hard on everyone. What the F..!

What just happened?! He was just saying goodbye to the babies, now there's blood everywhere. Get the fuck off of my kids. Shit, he shot me, again and again. Well, there are three more left in his gun. He's going to have to use them on me before he can touch another one of my babies. The chamber is empty. There's no new burning, only clicks when he pulls the trigger. I made it. He said I wasn't going to make it this time. I MADE IT! I MADE IT!

Mariah Clare LIVED through a horrible attack like the one above at the hands of her ex-husband (ksat). During the attack, he killed their 11-month-old daughter and critically injured their 2-year-old daughter. There were other children in the home during the attack that escaped assault by that guy. Evidence shows "that access to a gun makes it five times more likely that a woman will die at the hands of an abusive partner" (McFadden). In the words of Mariah Clare: "I want justice for my kids. This can't happen to people!"

"No matter how we identify, we all understand the value of what it means to be safe in our communities. Gun violence prevention policies should be connected to a shared sense of safety for all communities" (Barry).

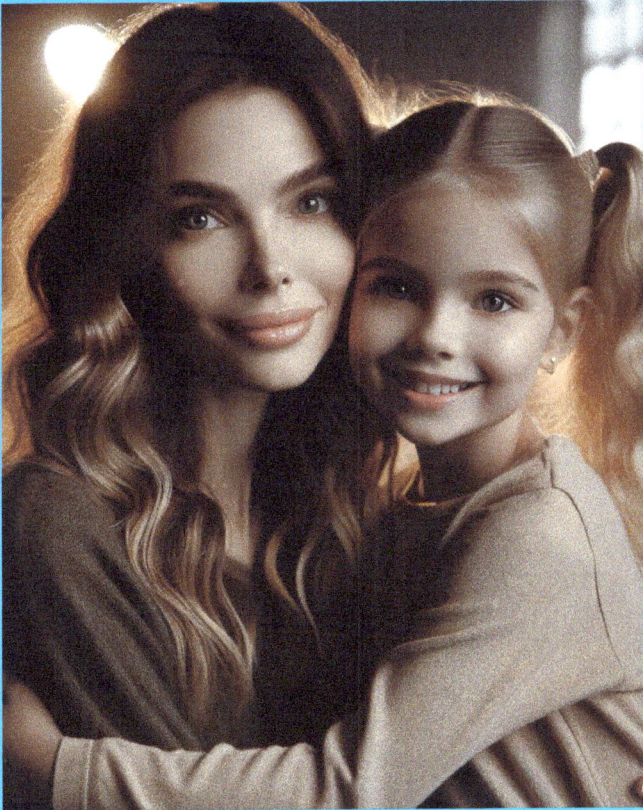

Activity: Debrief & Doodle

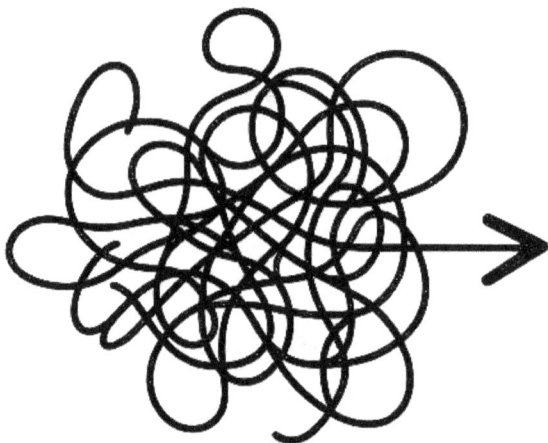

Untangling Chaos

Take a Big Breath In ...

BLOW

It Out 3 ... 2 ... 1

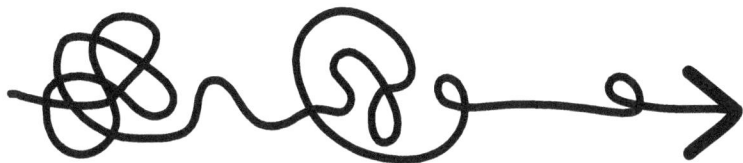

*Prolonged fear and anxiety keep our bodies' "fight or flight" response fired up. Overtime our bodies have difficulty maintaining a continuous flame (YoungMinds). The deep breathing helps our body pause and process the chaos around us (Russo, Macmillan).

How Did We Get Here?

Since the organization of the United States, Black, Indigenous, People of Color (BIPOC) and low-income people have lived in conditions that amplified health disparities. Segregation, redlining, and othering have contributed to these communities of people living near more environmental pollutants.

Dr. Robert D. Bullard's research highlights the patterns of hazardous waste sites and industrial pollution to excessively high levels of cancer, asthma, and other illnesses among vulnerable communities (Funes, MtSt/Pro, Long). These inequities add up over time to wear down the bodies of marginalized communities. Professionally, this wear and tear is known as allostatic load, and it manifests as poor health among people that bare this stress (Geronimus).

We know these gaps only widen during times of despair and crisis (Drake). The COVID Pandemic pulled back the curtain to a mountain of despair.

Repeatedly, communities experience significant emotional and mental trauma during times of crisis (RAND, SAMSHA T, Long). Hurricanes, massive snowstorms and earthquakes often permanently disrupt socially vulnerable (poor and working-class) communities (SPLC).

Hurricane Katrina is a gut-wrenching example of this devastation (Webster). Medical disasters impact vulnerable communities similarly to environmental disasters. BIPOC and Latinx people have carried the brunt of death and disability at the onset the COVID-19 (SARS-CoV-2) pandemic within the U.S. (Long, EJI).

Our society's worst nightmares came to life during the height of the pandemic. Rationing of medical care and allocating limited resources came into light among many states and hospital systems through the activation of "Crisis Standards of Care" (technical name for medical disaster policy) (SAEM).

Thus a decision of value, based on the health and longevity (expectancy) of each person that presented for care during times of limited resources came under review. There is concern that many of these horrors will re-appear with each natural or man-made disaster, and the people on the margins of making it will repeatedly be vulnerable and retraumatized.

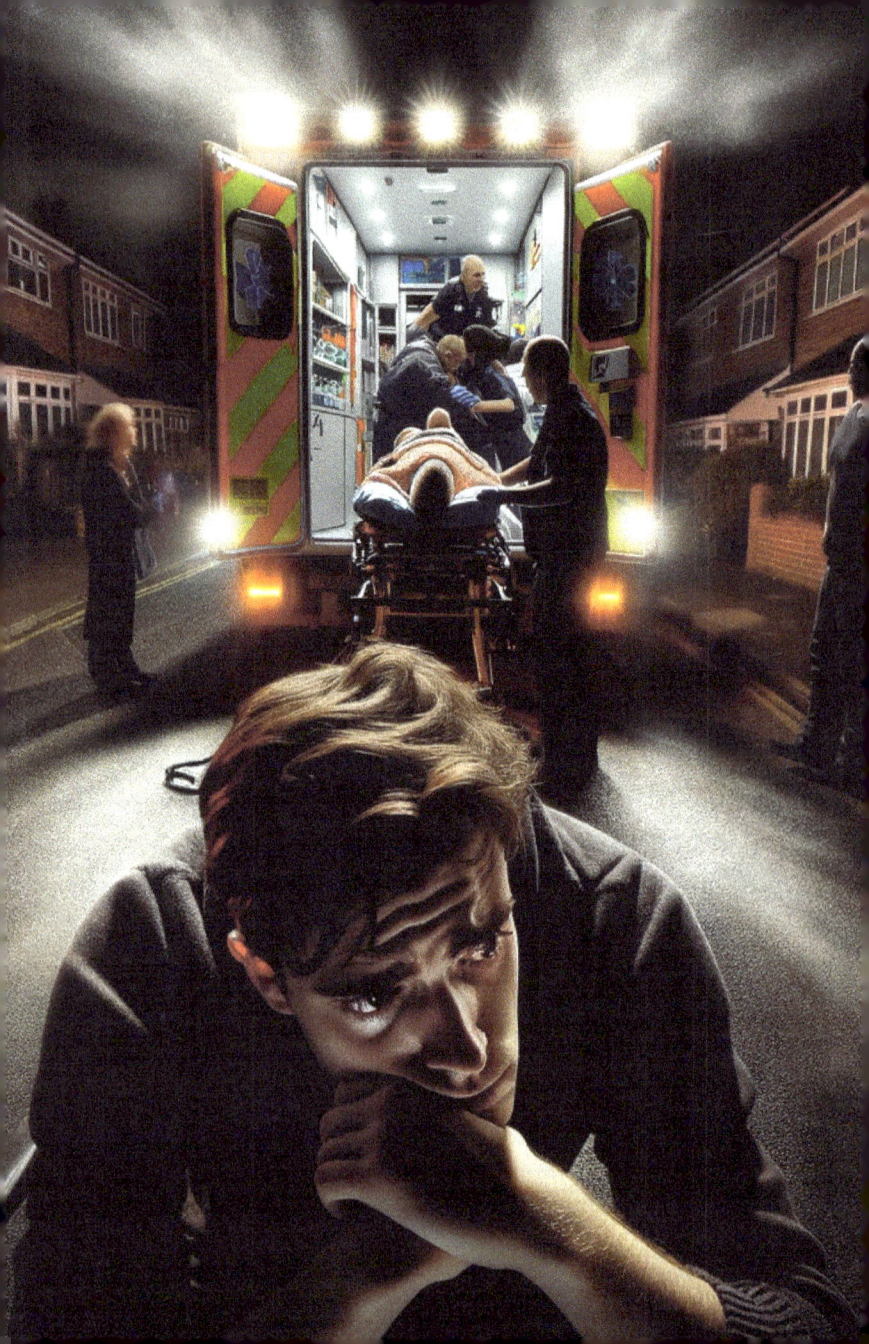

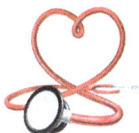

Chapter 8

Overdone By the Overdose
(SUBSTANCE USE DISORDER/ OPIOID EPIDEMIC)

Compassionate Letter

Oh Partner, I will tell you again. Your roommate said that you got home after the party, and something didn't seem right. You told her that you were going to sleep it off on the couch.

After her shower, she checked on you and you were purple, almost blue. She tried to shake you; you didn't respond. She called 9-1-1. When the paramedics came, they gave you naloxone or Narcan®, and you woke up somewhat. The rescue squad hurried as fast as they could to get you here.

You have nearly stopped breathing a few times since then, to the point that we've needed to give you oxygen and more naloxone just to keep from putting you on life support with a breathing tube. I understand that you want to get out of here as soon as possible. I am scared for you that the long-acting opioid drug isn't totally out of your system yet. The synthetics (narcotics) are more and more powerful each day.

We've seen a spike in the number of overdoses recently. I am thankful that your roommate checked on you, as you were on the train of death. You lived this time because you were not alone, and the rescue squad had naloxone at the ready. So many people, particularly those that take pills or drugs alone, don't pull through such an accident.

Kindred, we've now reached the end of your 6- to 8-hour observation period. You're alert and breathing by yourself now. Keep this naloxone with you and call 9-1-1 right away, if anyone you know uses it. Naloxone only lasts a short while, so they could stop breathing again. Every state in the country has approved the pharmacies and pharmacists to prescribe and dispense naloxone to anyone. Some even have it available over the counter, where you can just pick it up off the shelf (Saunders). Remember, be careful. There are no do-overs in the dope game!

Down to Earth explanation

Opioids (e.g., oxy, percs, dope, heroin, fentanyl, dilaudid, and other pain pills) suppress the brain's functions of alertness and breathing. Significant doses of opioids tell the body to stop breathing all together. This absence of oxygen triggers lung (pulmonary) then heart (cardiac) arrest. If not captured in time, this can lead to death.

As your body becomes accustomedo of opioids, it develops a tolerance to the starting doses/amounts of opioids ingested. Over time, larger amounts of opioids are needed to get the same high. Thus, people start to use more frequently or larger amounts. Such a pattern becomes a chronic cycle of disease. Extreme caution is needed after someone takes a break from using opioids because tolerance declines. Thus, if someone takes a dose of opioids equal to what they used before a period of abstinence (e.g., rehab), they could die from overdose. Their body is no longer accustomed to the higher doses of opioids (Kesten).

Care Considerations

Opioid reversal medication, naloxone (brand name- Narcan®), immediately reverses opioid effects on the body. It only lasts a few minutes. Thus, frequent doses of the medication are needed to support breathing until the opioids wear off. Opioid blockers (buprenorphine/ naltrexone) offer additional support with opioid use disorder. Methadone, a very slow-release opioid, can also be used to taper off opioids (NIDA). In the best scenarios the addiction treatment medications are used with counseling, behavioral therapy and social support. This combination of tools is called Medication-Assisted Treatment. Many hospitals offer patients the ability to start medication-assisted treatment for substance use disorder at the time of an overdose. In overdose cases when people come in alive and are not able to breath by themselves, oxygen and life support are provided until their bodies are able to breathe independently again. Critical care (ICU level care) is needed until the overdose wears off and people can breathe by themselves again.

Extreme patience, support and caution are needed with this chronic disease. Many people will undergo cycles of opioid use, abstinence, then relapse (Kesten). There is hope for an opioid-free life with great support.

U.S. Quick Facts

Opioid Use Observations

Opioid Deaths

• #1 cause of accidental death in the U.S. from opioid containing substances.

• The most common age range of opioid death patients is 25-34 years old.

• People 55+ years old are a rapidly growing cohort of opioid overdose deaths.

• Many people feel that opioid addiction is a private matter and often do not seek care.

Pearls for Further Explanation

• Si los labios son azules y ellos no se respira bien, **Llame 9-1-1** por el telephone o cellular.

• If someone has **blue lips and is not breathing well, call 9-1-1.**

• A prescription for overdose reversal medication (naloxone) is not needed (Fortier). Each of the 50 states has a standing order to dispense naloxone

(GoodRx).

• "Since 2015, the United States has seen a historic decline in life expectancy, in large part driven by the opioid epidemic and then the COVID-19 pandemic" (Klobucista). A substantial number of opioid over-doses are preventable.

Opioid Use

• Our bodies develop a physical and chemical dependence on opioids after more than 3-5 days of use (AARI).

• Opioids are commonly found in prescription pain medication (SAMHSA M).

• Synthetic opioids are often used to extend the strength or amplify pain pills, heroin, cocaine, or weed/marijuana (Gallagher).

Treatment

• **Discrete and supportive treatment options are available for substance use disorders.**

• Medications when used with supportive mental health therapy and social services have the greatest chance of opioid use recovery.

• This approach is known as Medication-Assisted Therapy (MAT).

• There are tremendous improvements to quality of life and financial incentives in receiving "evidence-based care" for opioid use disorder (Pew MAT).

• Text your zip code to 435748 (HELP4U). Help is available every hour of every day in multiple languages per SAMHSA.

• **No one is perfect. Many people will have to go through cycles of opioid use and abstinence.**

RX FOR SELF-ADVOCACY

Questions to Ask About Opioid Overdose Encounters:

• Is there a chance I could die, if I use (opioids) again? Yes, there is a very real chance that each time an opioid is used in a dose too high for the body or in combination with other drugs or alcohol, death can result.

• Do I need a prescription to get naloxone (Narcan®)? No, all 50 U.S. states, Puerto Rico and Washington, D. C. have it available at the pharmacy without a prescription (LAPPA). Some schools, libraries and community centers have naloxone available to give to the public (Good Rx, LAPPA).

•Where can I go to get help with not using? SAMHSA's National Helpline, 1-800-662-HELP (4357) or TTY: 1-800-487-4889. Text your zip code to 435748 (HELP4U). Help is available every hour of every day in multiple languages (SAMHSA).

Didn't I See That in the News?

"Mr. Addiction, you thought you had the final say. Well, this mama is telling you, no way!" Words spoken by a heart torn mother, Maryann Kordoski, on a day of education and remembrance of her two adult children taken by overdoses. Her pain from the loss of two children 15 months apart both from overdoses is unimaginable. Her strength to teach others through her pain is heroic.

Unfortunately, there are many other hero mothers, fathers, brothers, sisters, friends, partners, and children who are trying to figure out a new way forward. Sixty-six percent of U.S. adults "have been impacted by addiction, either personally or within their family" (Sparks). One in 10 U.S. adults have had a loved one die from a drug overdose (McPhillips, Sparks). In 2022 alone, almost 110,000 vibrant lives were lost due to overdoses. That's more people than some entire cities. So many of these vibrant lives could not find or access addiction treatment services (McPhillips). Now that we know that overdoses are not "just their problem," collectively we can support wholistic addiction and overdose treatment efforts to see the humanity of people who struggle with addiction and overdose. It cuts across all races, all classes and zip codes. (Sparks).

These struggles engulf the mental and financial health of family/friends/partners of those who struggle with excess use and abuse of drugs and alcohol. Truly, the person who struggles with substance use disorder does not struggle alone. Maybe we could consider treatment and support as a journey not to take alone.

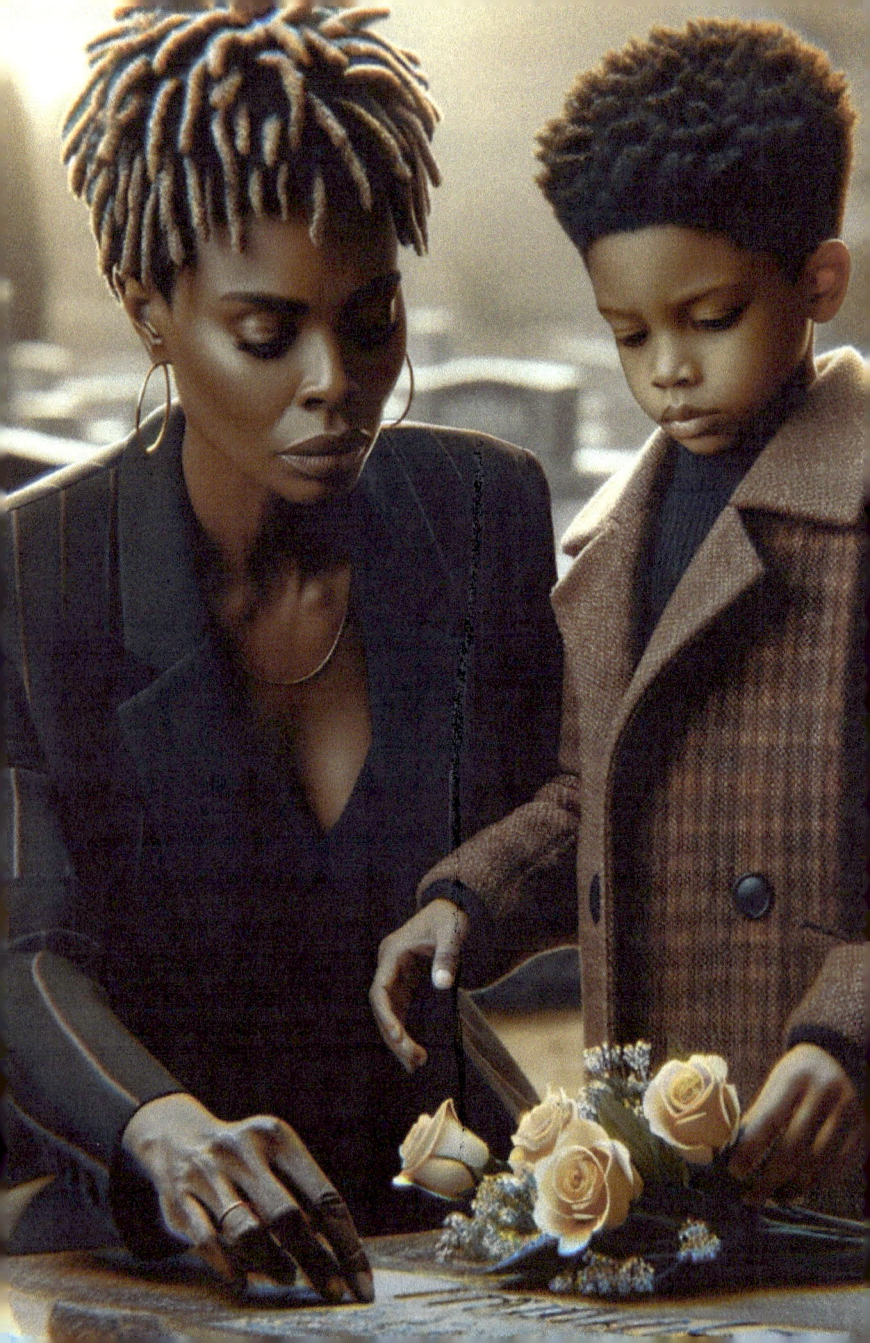

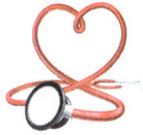

Chapter 9

COVID-19: is That Still a Thing?
(SARS-CoV-2)

Compassionate Letter

Am I breathing? Is this real. This is no dream. In the waiting room, there is a woman just sobbing, she's sobbing, sobbing so uncontrollably.

I say: Kindred, I know your heart is ripped apart right now. My heart is torn up, too. I put on the face of compassion and try not to break out into tears, as I tell you that your loved one has passed away from this life.

All she can say is: I never had a chance to say good-bye, I never had a chance to say goodbye. The wailing chorus continues for a few minutes more.

Kindred, I understand that the pandemic has taken your routine and freedom. And now I must tell you it has taken your parent. Yes, I will say it again, as it is so unbelievable. You saw him through the window of his nursing home every day for the last month. You knew in your heart that today, something seemed different. That little tickle in his throat had sunk lower into the lungs, and the cough had become almost constant.

I understand that your mind races and wonders, if the facility truly did right by your loved one. I hear you! I assure you; you did the right thing to encourage him to get checked out. No, this is not the flu. It's magnitudes worse. COVID-19 is predictable chaos. I know you wanted to be here with him during his evaluation and final moments. I know the video call just isn't the same. We just don't have enough protective equipment to keep staff and families safe from this thing.

Would it help to call a chaplain? Yes! Ok, the chaplain will be here soon. I'll make a mental note to ask the chaplain to pray for me after they meet with your family. I'm not sure how much longer I can go on like this. Maybe if I have a few drinks tonight, tomorrow will be better. And the nightmare of COVID-19 will be one day closer to ending.

Down to Earth Explanation
COVID-19 Disease & SARS-CoV-2 Germ

COVID-19 disease is caused by a very contagious virus that is passed around through the secretions of our coughs, sneezes and vocalizations (e.g., talking, singing, cheering, yelling) (EPA, CDC SB). The specific virus that causes COVID-19 is the "coronavirus disease SARS-CoV-2" (CDC B). This was first reported anywhere in the world during December 2019 (CDC B).

These SARS-CoV-2 germs can float in the air for 2-3 hours (EPA, CDC SB) and last on surfaces for up to 3 days (CDC SB). The COVID-19 germs gain entry into our bodies through the moist surfaces of our eyes, nose and mouth. This germ is hard to shake off or avoid because it has extra sticking power to our cells. Its "spiked proteins" cling so tightly and help the germ get inside our bodies (Henry Ford, Thorne).

Face masks help capture and reduce the amount of virus in the air and on surfaces. Quality masks made of the correct materials help reduce the chance of spreading the germs to other people. Frequent hand-washing can minimize the chance of you contaminating yourself after touching objects that other people (possibly infected) have used. An acute COVID infection typically shows up with diarrhea, cough, congestion, fever, body aches 2-14 days after exposure to the germ (CDC C19). COVID infection typically lasts 1–2 weeks (WHO C). More severe forms of the infection can cause difficulty breathing, low oxygen levels, blue/purple coloring to the lips, confusion, chest pain or worse (WHO C).

A noticeable number of people go on to develop Long COVID. Typically, this presents as continued COVID symptoms 4 weeks after the initial infection. "Long COVID occurs more often in people who had severe COVID-19 illness, but anyone who has been infected with the virus that causes COVID-19 can experience it" (CDC LC).

Each time a person is infected with the COVID-19 virus, there is a risk of the infection progressing to Long COVID (CDC LC). The duration of Long COVID is variable, with a substantial number of children (Jiang) and adults (Burns) having symptoms months beyond the initial infection. COVID can rob people of their lives. The U.S. comprises just over 4% of all the people in the world (US Census, worldmeter) and has the highest number of covid infections and deaths. The U.S. far exceeds other countries in the number of people that have died from COVID (WHO D). This is an unfortunate title to hold, particularly as a well-resourced country.

Care Considerations

Initially, there were no specific treatments for COVID-19. Medical professionals did what they could to support people through the hard and critical times. This meant giving oxygen, pressor medications to keep blood pressure up, steroids, and life support with breathing tubes to the lungs when the pandemic started.

Over time therapies targeted at the COVID-19 virus were developed. These anti-virals and monoclononal antibiodies are medications that reduced the chance of death and severe disability. Which targeted COVID medicines used depends on the severity of the ill- ness, patient hospitalization status, and the particular viral variant causing illness. The greatest weapons came less than one year (December 2021) into this war. The COVID-19 updated vaccines reduce the chance of getting admitted into the overstretched hospitals or dying from COVID.

Today, teams of doctors and providers work together in Long COVID centers to give specialized treatment to people who suffer with the lingering effects of COVID.

U.S. Quick Facts

COVID-19 Disease

(Is Short for Coronavirus Disease 2019)
Caused by the viral germ named SARS-CoV-2
(CDC B).

• This new germ is now the **#4 Cause of Death in U.S.** (Ahmad).

• "In 2020, COVID-19 became the third leading cause of death, surpassing all other causes except heart disease and cancer" (Johnson, CDC LD)

• "Half of all states and nearly three quarters of all counties experienced more deaths than births — known as natural decrease — in the 2021 estimates year"(Johnson).

• COVID-19 is not just a big city problem. It has dramatically decreased the average lifespan of Americans, eliminating decades of public health gains (Klobucista).

Pearls for Further Explanation

Consider these tips to make safer surroundings and reduce risk of catching COVID.

• "**Avoid the 3Cs**: spaces that are **C**losed, **C**rowded or involve **C**lose contact.

• Meet people outside. Outdoor gatherings are safer than indoor ones, particularly if indoor spaces are small and without outdoor air coming in.

• If you can't avoid crowded or indoor settings, take these precautions:
  - **Open a window** to increase the amount of natural ventilation when indoors.
  - **Wear a mask** (WHO C).

What is **Long COVID (Post COVID)?**
Survivor Corps has information about Post Covid/ Long Covid Care Centers and other tips:

https://www.survivorcorps.com/long-covid-faqs

Long Covid Support Groups

• Ask your Health Care Provider for a referral.

• Consider social media: Facebook, Instagram, Tik Tok, X formerly Twitter.

• Groups like Survivor Corps with their Family/ Caregiver supports: https://www.survivorcorps. com/homecare

• Testimonial from COVID Survivor: Dr. Margot Gage Witvliet -TEDx Mile High Talk https://www.youtube.com/watch?v=4LX_JRHZdkl

Families of those with COVID

• Survivor Corps Family/Caregiver supports: https://www.survivorcorps.com/homecare

• Caring for People with Post-COVID Conditions: https://www.cdc.gov/coronavirus/2019-ncov/long-term-effects/care-post-covid.html

• Preparing for Appointments for Post-COVID Conditions: https://www.cdc.gov/coronavirus/2019-ncov/long-term-effects/post-covid-appointment/index.html (CDC LC)

Resources

• Common Questions about COVID-19 and Indoor Air Answered by the EPA: https://www.epa.gov/coronavirus/frequent-questions-about-indoor-air-and-coronavirus-covid-19

• **To find COVID-19 vaccine locations near you:** Search vaccines.gov, text your ZIP code to 438829, or call 1-800-232-0233 (CDC Covid Treatment Med)

• **Need help finding a place to get medication?** Call 1-800-232-0233 (TTY 888-720-7489) https://covid-19-test-to-treat-locator-dhhs.hub.arcgis.com/ (ASPR Get Meds)

Transmission

• The main way to contract COVID is by coming in contact with an infected person's airway (pathway from mouth/nose to lungs) secretions via droplets and aerosols (CDC SB).

• COVID virus can live indoors on surfaces of plastic and stainless steel for up to 3 days (van Doremalen).

• Enclosed spaces/indoor places are high risk for spreading COVID germs (CDC SB EPA).

• Masks, routine surface cleaning and good hand washing reduce the spread of the germs (CDC SB).

Prevention

• Proper usage of masks, quality handwashing, physical distancing between people, and vaccinations are very effective at reducing the spread of the COVID germ.

• People with certain health conditions (e.g., pregnancy, chemotherapy use) that increase the risk of complications from COVID-19 should strongly consider vaccination against the virus to reduce severe disease or death. People with weakened immune system may need additional vaccinations for ideal protection (CDC B).

• Everyone else is strongly encouraged to get the vaccine if there are no severe allergic reactions to the components, a COVID vaccine is available to you or you have no fever or active COVID infection (WHO C).

• Combining prevention measures creates the greatest protection against catching the COVID-19 disease.

• COVID-19 COUNTY CHECK to see how hospital admissions are trending: https://www.cdc.gov/coronavirus/2019-ncov/your-health/covid-by-county.html

• Consider increasing preventative measures when hospital admissions start to rise.

• COVID Global Activity per World Health Organization: https://covid19.who.int/

• To find COVID-19 vaccine locations near you: Search vaccines.gov, text your ZIP code to 438829, or call 1-800-232-0233 (CDC Covid Treatment Med).

Treatment

• Mild cases: may be treated with rest and supportive care.

• Moderate cases: steroids, oxygen, anti-virals, blood thinning medications, +/- monoclonantibodies.

• Severe cases: intensive care unit (ICU) therapies and interventions to maintain oxygenation and blood pressure in addition to moderate treatments. **"Don't delay: Treatment must be started within days of when you first develop symptoms to be effective"** (CDC Covid Treatment Medications).

Scientists are actively searching for treatments for COVID-19; as more evidence is gathered, more tailored therapies can be created.*

• **FDA Approved Therapies:**
- Veklury (remdesivir)
- Paxlovid (nirmatrelvir/ritonavir) (FDA)

• **Previously the FDA extended Emergency Use Authorization (EUA)** for other preventative and treatment therapies during time of crisis (EUA).

Resources:
• "If you have questions about any medication, contact the FDA's Division of Drug Information at 301-796-3400 or druginfo@fda.hhs.gov" (FDA).

• **Need help finding a place to get medication or visit?** Call 1-800-232-0233 (TTY 888-720-7489) https://covid-19-test-to-treat-locator-dhhs.hub.arcgis.com/ (ASPR Get Meds)

Children Whose Parent or Caregiver Died From COVID

• **299,275 children younger than 18 have been orphaned due to COVID-19 between January 2020 through June 2023. ++**

• Indigenous children lost the most caregivers at 4 times the rate of White Children (Global Ref).

• **These children have survived at least one ACE (adverse childhood experience) and possibly more.**

• This traumatic event increases the risk of mental health problems, poorer school performance and increase for chronic health conditions and abuse.

• Comprehensive emotional, mental, social and often financial support can help reduce the trauma impact from the loss of a parent/caregiver and assist the children with healthy relationship skills (Slomski).

Resources:

• **Runaway or Homeless Youth** Phone: 1-800-RUNAWAY (1-800-786-2929) or Text: 66008

- **Childhelp® National Child Abuse Hotline** at 1-800-4-A-CHILD (1-800-422-4453) to report suspected abuse.

- **National Childhood Traumatic Stress Network** for information and resources to address different traumas (bullying, sex trafficking, crime): https://www.nctsn.org/what-is-child-trauma/trauma-types

*This list is not exhaustive and each patient's care plan is tailored to their unique needs.

++The number of orphaned children due to COVID grows each day in the U.S. and around the world. For current information go to the Global Reference Group on Children Affected by COVID-19 website: https://imperialcollegelondon.github.io/orphanhood_USA/.

RX FOR SELF-ADVOCACY

Questions to Ask About COVID-19 Encounters:

• What are my oxygen levels? Please note that some people with darker skin color have a blood sample oxygen level (aka arterial blood gas) lower than what the noninvasive finger pulse ox demonstrates. **Always seek/provide care based on how the patient feels** "https://hms.harvard.edu/news/skin-tone-pulse-oximetry" (HMS, Gottlieb).

• How do I monitor my oxygen levels at home?

• When should I come back to the hospital for care?

• What is the best evidence-based care available for COVID-19 for someone with my health conditions?

• What is the best science today for treatment?

• I'm so concerned that something is wrong. I'm not getting better. It's been over a month now. What Long COVID resources are available?

Didn't I See That in the News?

Inspired by Dr. Margot Gage Witvliet

What! No, I'm not addicted to drugs. I'm no seeker. I've never felt pain like this before. I had two kids by natural childbirth and still never felt this bad. Something is not right. This is not just a cold. I'll try again. I'll use my best professional voice.

Don't they know I'm a doctor. WTF! Do I have to get ignorant to get some care. Something is not right. I just know it. Sad to say that Dr. Gage Wiltvliet's experience in fighting to get treatment is not isolated.

Several high-profile, exceptionally educated women of color have spoken out about the disregard they experienced in seeking medical care for COVID-like symptoms. For at least one of these women, Dr. Susan Moore, the disregard likely took her life (Eligon, Miller).

COVID is swift. First it took our Elders, then our healthcare workers, and our youthful essential workers. Once it got on our blocks, dissemination occurred. There was no town, county or city left unscarred by COVID-19. Our nation's life expectancy has fallen by the most it has in 100 years due to COVID (Johnson).

Are we looking at the beginning of a horrible squeal or an evil time clock of reversal with each COVID surge?

The at least 1.1 million Americans who lost their lives to COVID-19 had meaning beyond their lives (WHO, CDC Data). Many were police officers, EMS workers, teachers, nurses, cashiers. Their families and communities mourn their deaths and loss of their talents. Collectively as a country, we see this as losses in public health and mental health measures. Maybe more concerningly, educational standings as a nation have taken a mighty blow.

We know of the 1.1 million American lives lost from COVID. How many of these were unnecessary or could have been avoided had they had valid information (not misinformation), or if they could have accessed high-quality care?

No one is above COVID and the havoc it brings. Everyone can use their power to protect themselves from this virus that is never going away. It is possible to catch covid multiple times, as it is an ever-changing virus (Reed). It helps to have a global perspective of how other countries are living with COVID. Other countries consistently prioritize the most vulnerable and high risk amongst them to vaccinate to reduce hospitalizations and death. With limited resources and limited downtime for the most youthful, healthy portions of their communities, efforts are being placed on vaccinating people older than 65 years in the early phases of vaccine roll out.

It is hoped that we, society, come away from a scarcity mindset surrounding vaccinations and can have them available for all who want them. Though the youthful and the healthy are deferred in the initial rounds of vaccinations, many of these folks are in close contact with elders and the immunocompromised. Which means the "healthy" are at risk of bringing the virus home to those they love who may not have a healthy immune system to fight germs.

Every time we catch COVID, the risk of complications and Long COVID lurch for adults and children alike (Kavanagh, O'Bier). The CDC noted in 2022 that 1.3% of children and 6.9% of adults had Long COVID (CDC LC). "Long COVID occurs more often in people who had severe COVID-19 illness, but anyone who has been infected with the virus that causes COVID-19 can experience it" (CDC LC). Long COVID should be considered to be present if new or recurring COVID symptoms present 4 weeks after the initial infection (CDC LC). Those things that just won't go away should be evaluated, particularly by Long COVID clinics and specialists.

It seems that COVID will be here with us indefinitely. This is a chance for us to see and hear one another to create a better future.

> "I was not treated with dignity,"
> —Dr. Margot Gage Witvliet

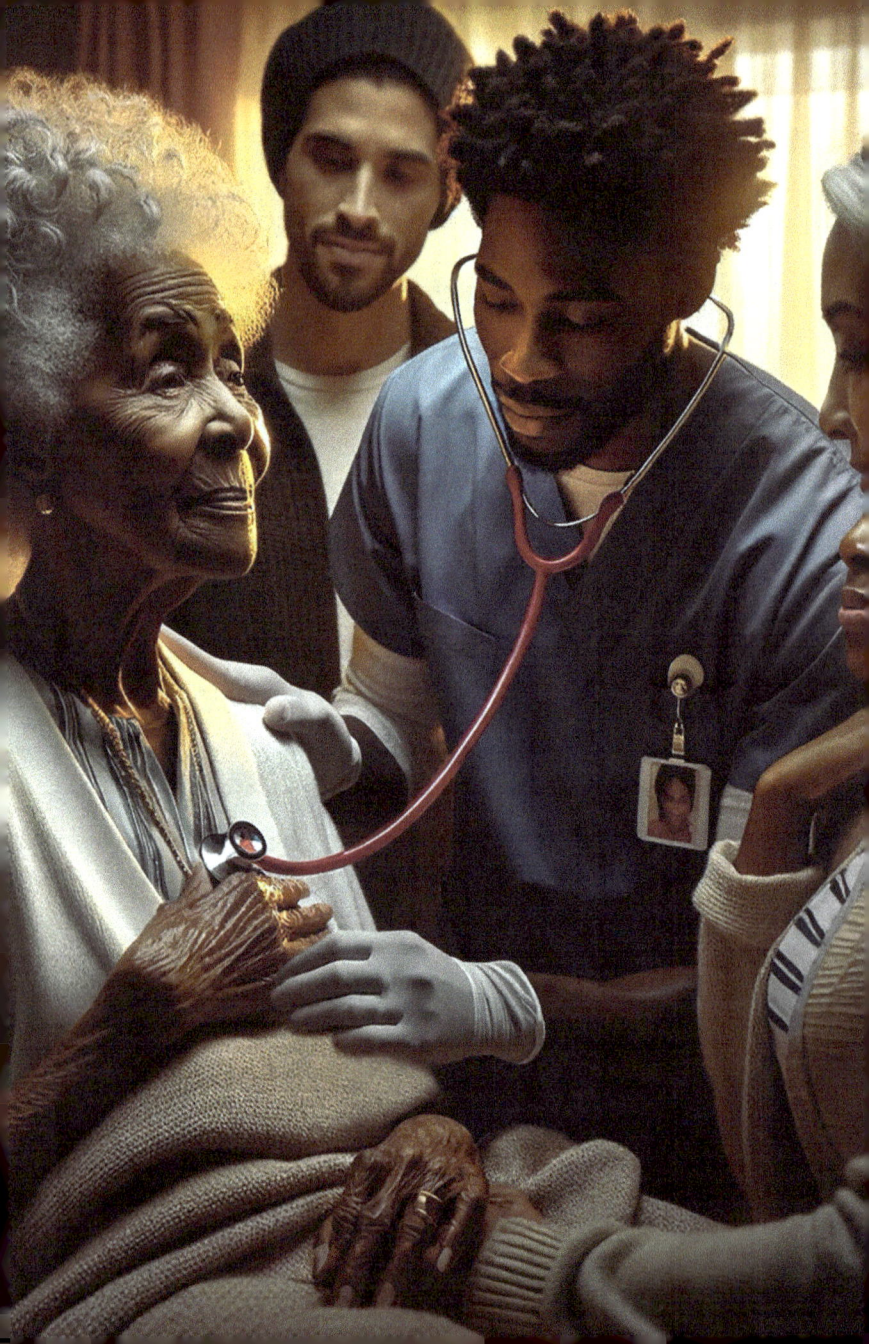

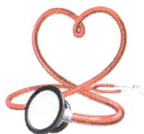

Chapter 10

End of Life is Not the End of Hope

Compassionate Letter

Beloved, I am happy to take care of you. Our job is to support you and your wishes. I understand this has been a long journey with this terminal disease. You have earned the right to express your life how you see fit. Now, what do you need? What do you want? Umm, I'll get right on it.

Is it the weakness or the pain that has you most un-comfortable? Ok, we will start with great medicine for pain control. You have options for how this journey will play out. I know it feels that things have been out of your control. Our job is to give you honor and control now.

It is obvious that your greatest wish is to care for your family more than yourself. You can see how hard this transition is for them. You don't have to carry this worry alone. We can have our spiritual care team and grief counselors support you and your family during this time.

Now that the pain is better controlled, I'm so glad you have a few moments to think more clearly. I understand that this has been your biggest fight, and it feels like you have nothing left. You are brave and are giving an excellent fight. You know this "thing" won't go away, AND it doesn't have to win. You are the conductor of this orchestra. Together our team can help make something beautiful out of this. Who would you like present? How is your pain? The waves are coming closer. We will keep up with it. Have you thought of words to leave your family with? How do you want them to celebrate the journey of life that you are taking?

Now the room is quiet, your loves are all around. They see your peace and thank you for not letting them do this alone. Our team will give you private time. We'll be just outside the room.

You breathe in this moment, your loves at your side. You close your eyes and take your flight. It has been an honor to respectfully care for you. May you have peace with this journey.

Down to Earth explanation

We will all meet death one day. The hope is that it will find each of us after a full and rich life.

Approaching death is a time of the great unknown. It does not have to be traveled from a powerless position. You have choices along the way. You can fight a terminal illness on your terms. There are kind hearts who can help you make your wishes known. How will you embrace this transition to create future memories of peace and hope for your family? What meaning will you make in this moment? What loving light will you leave to the world?

Care Considerations

How can we help you transition from this earth with the dignity you deserve?

The goal is to help you "live the best life you can, and use your time for what's most important to you" (ACS E). It's okay to take some time to get really clear about what is important to you. It often helps to speak with a trained counselor to help you process what you feel and organize your thoughts. Including your loved ones in your thought process could be helpful, as well. Participating in communities of support or spiritual practice may help calm your mind and provide hope. These acts will only help you fine tune your goals and actions.

If you are lost and have no clue where to start, lean on your healthcare team right away. Your team of providers are likely aware of services that can help you manage your pain (palliation) or make the transition to death as comfortable as possible (hospice). Palliative care teams are dedicated to making treatment of terrible diseases less painful. They work together with you and your treating physicians to figure out how to ease the pain while fighting the disease. If there comes a time when "treatments" do not feel like a help, there can be a pivot to a Hospice Team to draw up a play for comfort and rest. Many services are available to you and those you love as death approaches up to one year after the transition for your family of origin or family of choice (HFA).

If you have been without a health care team for a while and have few connections, consider reaching out to the Hospice Foundation of America by calling toll free 800-854-3402. Their team is available during business hours and are on the Eastern Time zone. After getting connected to hospice services, many people and their families express a wish to have known about the services earlier (HFA). Studies even back up many families' gut feelings. The data demonstrates that "hospice care often is not started soon enough" (ACS H).

Remember, you are in control of how this journey will go. If hospice is something you change your mind about, that is okay. It is really okay. The goal is to live your life in a way that is in alignment with your beliefs and honors your presence. Sometimes, it's hard to know what you truly want until you can experience it for yourself. If you decide you would like to go back to hospice care, that is possible as well through the re-enrollment process.

Sometimes a change in scenery can be helpful and restorative, as well. There are respite care services designed just for this matter. You may decide to take a small break for a few hours or days at a care facility. Alternatively, you can arrange to have in-home respite services to allow your caregivers and/or family a chance to attend to their own appointments or just grab a break. Watching a loved one in a condition that is not quite their typical is hard for those that love them to see and experience. It is also, physically intense. Finding the balance that allows everyone involved in end-of-life care to give their best attention, time and love is the key. The goal is not to have anyone burn out and compromise their health or wellness during this journey. Your people love you very much. Sometimes they need a recharge to be their very best selves.

Oh, the money to pay for these things. You are concerned about all of the bills. I know it is stressful. Insurance (private or governmental), sliding scales, grants, donations (ACS P), charity care, financing are several options to get the services you wish for. Each team that provides care can help you understand the best way to receive services.

You are worthy of compassionate and respectful care through live and after death. Your wishes are important and can be very helpful if shared with those closest to you. Would you like to be celebrated with a home funeral after you have passed on? Are there certain ceremonies or rituals that are important to honor the body that you leave behind? Is it important that you have a green (or natural) burial or no burial at all? You don't have to have the answers right away. It may take some time to truly reflect on what is important to you. The most important thing is that you do what feels right to you. You are worthy of a fuss. Our job is to help support you beyond the end.

"You matter because of who you are. You matter to the last moment of your life, and we will do all we can, not only to help you die peacefully, but also to live until you die."

–Dame Cicely Saunders (ACS P)

U.S. Quick Facts

End of Life Observations

Choice & Control

• 76.4 years of age is current life expectancy for people in the U.S. (CDC L).

• Life expectancy has plummeted since 2020 mostly due to COVID-19 (CDC LE).

• Indigenous people had the biggest drop in life expectancy in 2021, loosing 1.9 years.

• In 2021, the life expectancy of an Indigenous person was 65.2 years (CDC LE).

• "Despite being a top spender on health care, the United States ... sits well in the bottom half of" high-income countries for health outcomes and life expectancy (Klobuscista).

Pearls For Further Explanation

Resources:

• ACS: Coping with Emotions as You Near the End of Life: https://www.cancer.org/treatment/end-of-life-care/nearing-the-end-of-life/emotions.html

• Solidifying your wishes for end of life: Advanced Directives can make your desires known if you are unable to speak for yourself.

For help with setting up your Advanced Directives, contact your local Area Agency on Aging by calling 800-677-1116.

What is Palliative Care

• Palliative Care optimizes quality of life for patients while they undergo treatment for debilitating medical conditions.

• Focuses on lightening the load from the physical, emotional, and psychosocial tolls of illness on patients and their families.

• People with the following diagnoses benefit from palliative care: stroke, cancer, dementia, chronic obstructive pulmonary disease (COPD). People with other serious conditions can benefit from palliative care, as well (Feke).

Hospice

• The last several years have seen increasing numbers of people us hospice services: "1.61 million Medicare beneficiaries received hospice care in 2019" (Statista) and 1.72 million in 2020 (NPHCO F) for end of life care.

• People with the following diagnoses most often utilize hospice care services: Alzheimers Disease, Dementia, Parkinson's, and Cancer (NPHCO). Other end of life conditions are cared for, as well.

What is Hospice?

• "Hospice care provides compassionate care for people in the last phases of incurable disease so that they may live as fully and comfortably as possible … A team of professionals work together to manage symptoms so that a person's last days may be spent with dignity and quality, surrounded by their loved ones"(ACS H).

• Hospice Foundation of America: https://hospice-foundation.org/Hospice-Care/Hospice-Services

• "We never forget that behind the data points are people." "That's why the hospices across the country work tirelessly to provide person and family-centered, interdisciplinary care to help them during a time of great need" (NPHCO).

Burial Customs

- Death and burial preparations of the bodies of people that have passed on have strong cultural significance, centered in dignity and respect (Amanik, Fletcher).

- Traditional cemeteries for internment are not mandated.

- Private property burials may be possible (WPR).

- Regulations surrounding burial procedurals vary by state (WPR).

Caregiver Support/Tips

- **Care giving is hard.**
- It can be exponentially harder when caring for someone at the end of their life.

Resources

- "Encourage your loved one to make as many decisions as they can to maintain control in their life. As long as they are making safe decisions, let your loved one have the final say"...

- "Listen to your loved one and let them know that you hear what they are saying"....

- "Even if you disagree with the wishes your loved one expresses, respect their right to decide"...

• "**Create a peaceful atmosphere.** Sometimes words are unnecessary. Keep your loved one warm, clean and comfortable. Play soft music, as hearing is thought to be the last sense."

• Considerations for caregiver self-care: Listen to friends or family if they notice changes in your mood.

• Maintain contact with friends and family. Social isolation can increase emotional distress.

• Try to give yourself a half-hour to an hour each day outside the house.

• Remember to eat three meals every day. Even if the meals are small, they will give you energy to take care of your loved one.

• Drink water regularly.

• Try to get uninterrupted sleep (6–8 hours). This might require that you get some assistance in caring for your loved one at home (Cancer Care.)

RX FOR SELF-ADVOCACY

Questions to Ask About End-of-Life Care:

• How do I have control/power when everything seems awry?

• Will my partner/family be okay?

• What services (spiritual services/hospice) are available to them?

• How do I make my desires or wishes known?

• What if I can't talk for myself when the time comes?

• I love my family and have given my best. How do I not let myself or my family down?

Didn't I See That in the News?

"Perhaps nothing alleviates a dying person's fear of death more than love," per Sheldon Soloman (Horovitz). Folks who know death is imminently coming for them can be very unsettled.

Some seek for something in the physical to slow death down to gain one more day. Some realize that the burden they bear approaching death is unrelenting. However, experiencing compassion, kindness, and knowing that they've made an impact can help ease the transition.

Knowing that they have been seen and valued can bring peace and comfort that no money can buy.

"Everything can be taken from a man but one thing: the last of the human freedoms—to choose one's attitude in any given set of circumstances, to choose one's own way."
—V. Frankl

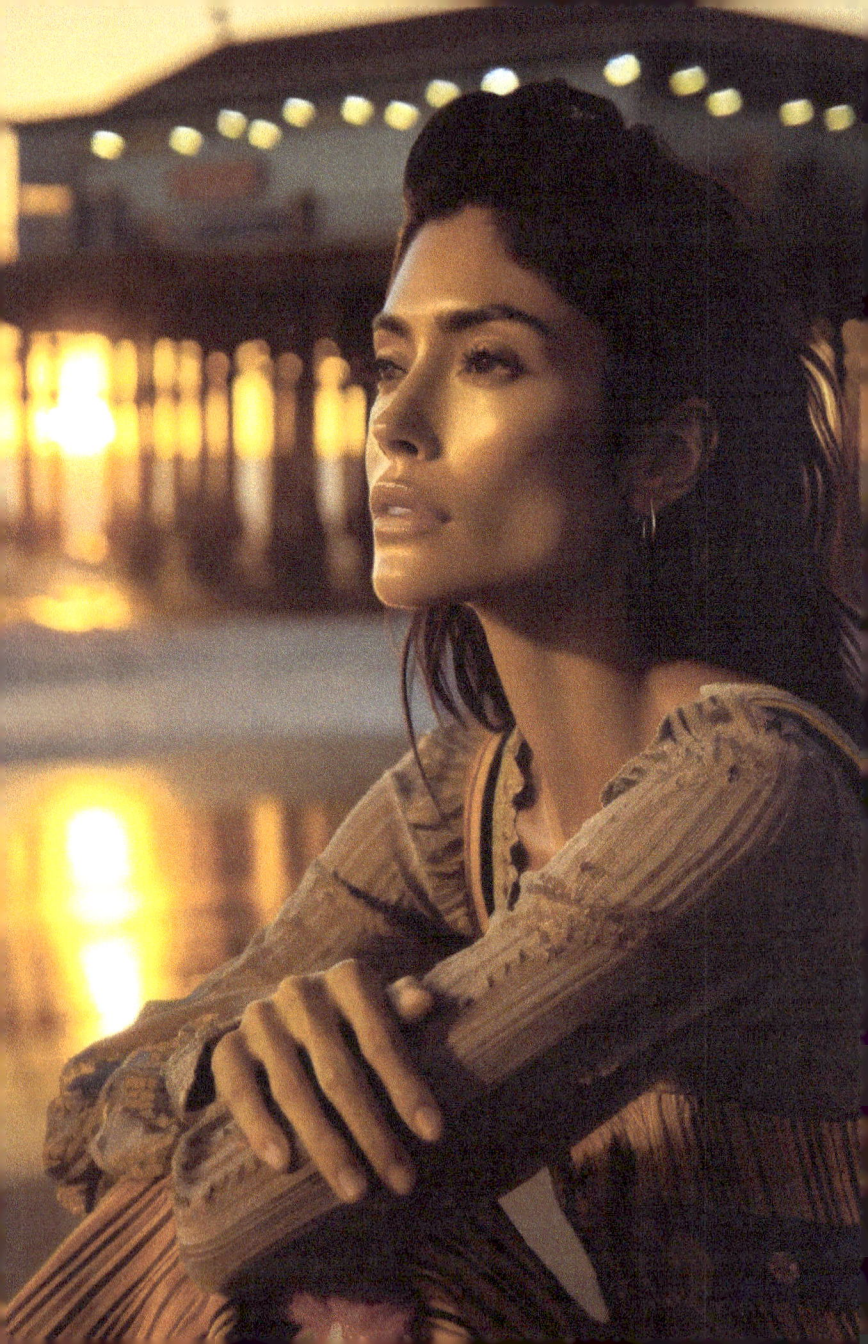

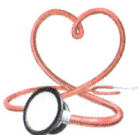

Chapter 11

The Power in Making Your Choices Known

Compassionate Letter

You are deserving of respect and compassion. It really doesn't matter what you've done in the past. We've all had less than perfect days. And as human beings, we are not perfect. It is hoped that we grow from each moment in which we were less than what we truly desired to be. We all have different starting points, and we all will have different endpoints. No matter how rough or rocky the start may be, you have the power to choose a different course. It is important that you sit with yourself and think about what are the things that are important to you. Is it coming and going, moving and shaking, or being still feeling the ocean's breeze hug your skin? These are the questions that first you should ask yourself <u>before</u> reaching out to other people.

Once you are clear on what brings you joy, it's okay to share those joys with those that you love dearest.
It can be helpful to have this talk when it seems like all is right in the world. When a critical or terminal illness comes, these conversations can be very difficult without some starting point.

It doesn't matter if you have one million dollars in your bank account or a no dollars account. Just know that the Love Letters To Patients® Community is here to support you. Each person, each voice has priceless value. Know that your voice has power and know that you are seen. You are contributing to a more respectful and compassionate world.

May you know that you are the greatest!

"I don't have to be who you want me to be;
I'm free to be who I want."

—*Muhammad Ali* (Ali Center)

Activity:

Doodle in power

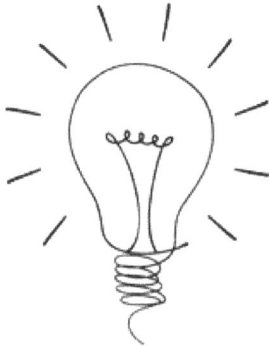

You are powerful.

You have the right to competent and dignified healthcare. *Give yourself sometime. When our brains and bodies are in overdrive, it's hard to think clearly (MacMillan). It takes 20-30 minutes for your body to reset after a really stressful event (Karmin). Doodling can help your body and mind return to a place of calm and relaxation (Neumann). How about you give it a go!

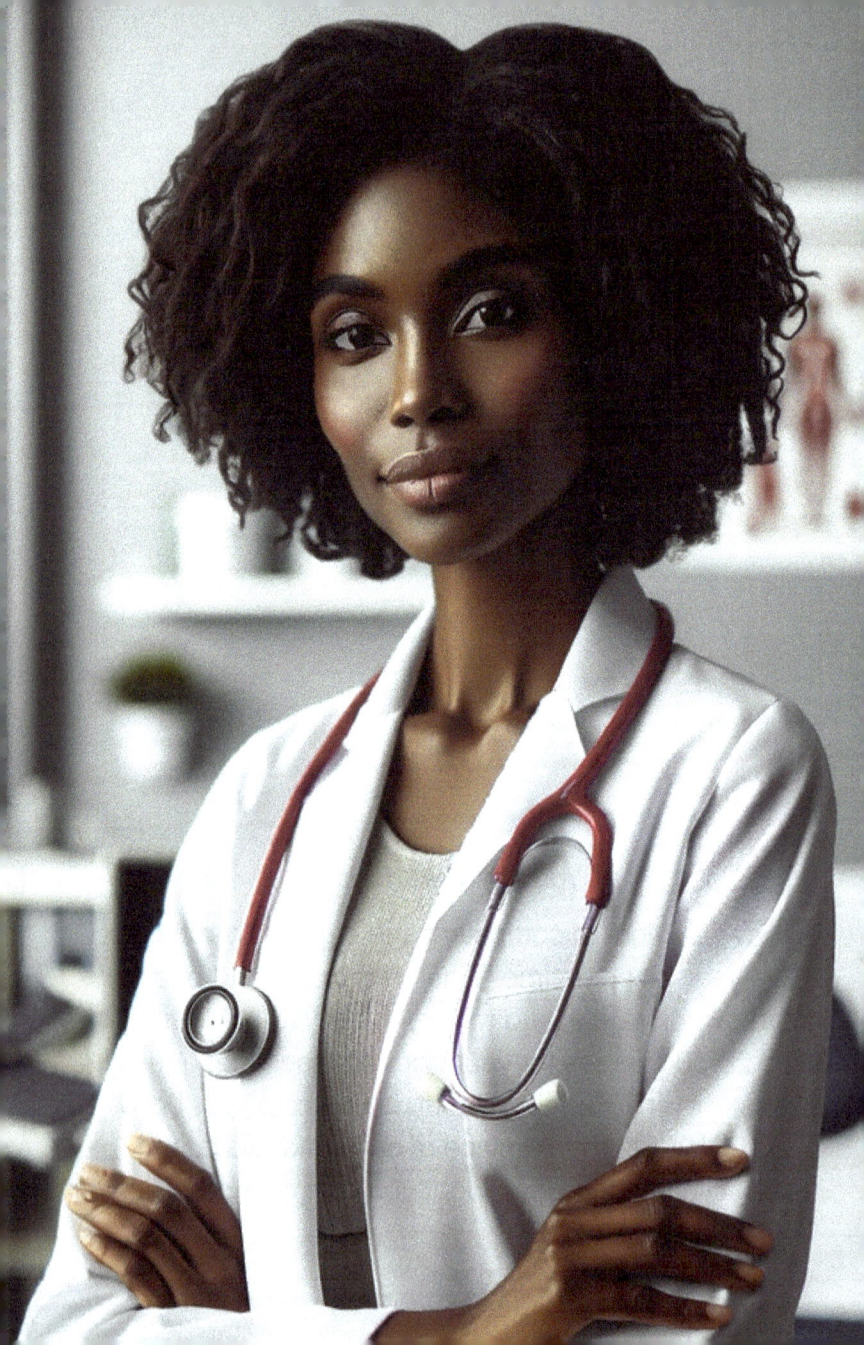

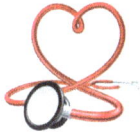

Chapter 12

RJ as an Rx for Hope

Restorative Justice

Restorative Justice (RJ) is a school of thought and a collection of practices that center people at the heart of harm, hurt, disagreement, or unrest with those that created the distress. The intention of the practices is to make wrongs right for the people and community that were harmed during an event and to reduce the harm from happening again. Each person engaged in the restorative process has equal worth and insight into the situation. Restorative justice equalizes power between all parties involved in a harmful/hurtful event in the process of acknowledging and repairing the hurts of a harmful event (Yazzie, Long, Karp, Kaba, Boyes-Watson, Jenkins).

Chief Justice Robert Yazzie has said that restorative justice eliminates the "vertical hierarchy" of power. This is the concept that decisions are wielded from high by an authority figure. The fact that each participant involved in a harmful event has input into the corrective action is known as "the horizontal justice model" in which "no person is above the other" (Yazzie).

Many Indigenous Communities and Restorative Justice Practitioners use circular seating arrangements during meetings with parties involved in a harmful event to facilitate conversation. "In a circle, there is no right or left, no beginning or end. Every point (or person) on the line on a circle looks to the same center as the focus. The circle is the symbol of Navajo justice because it is perfect, unbroken, and a simile of unity and oneness (Yazzie)." **Genuine respect for each person's perspective builds collective trust, enabling partnership and innovation to create solutions.**

RJ has the superpower of placing acts of harm within a bigger context for each party that was involved and the community that was impacted. It is context and circumstances that shaped the event. It is with a fuller understanding of the context from all vantage points that will create a full picture of the act of harm and shape solutions.

Blinding stakeholders to select portions of the context will remove the event(s) from within the context of the United States societal history. By omitting the complete picture, there is limited insight into the pattern of trauma from "racial injustice, genocide and segregation" (Davis) and patriarchy. **There is potential for creating more harm when decisions are made from an incomplete vantage point.** Limited contextual understanding perpetuates acts of harm against marginalized communities (Davis).

When a hurt occurs, be it from delayed diagnosis or death from medical mishap, it is of utmost importance that each participant's humanity is recognized. When people are "othered," it leads way to anger and hatred which eat away at people (Davis). Othering is a reflection of society's power dynamics (Akbulut), and its valuation of human worth. Over time, this leads way to the creation of marginalized communities. **Simply put, othering defines who belongs and who does not belong within the larger context of society** (Akbulut). When applied through a healthcare lens, there are "potential negative consequences (that) exist for human development, maintenance of self-esteem, and health promotion and restoration" (Canales).

It is very challenging to undergo such continuous stress without direct impact to self and community. Dr. Geronimus commented that: "Poor and nonpoor Black women had the highest and second highest probability of cumulative wear and tear on the body's systems" from trying to compensate for societal stressors (McEwen, Geronimus). This phenomenon of bearing the stress is known as allostatic load. When compared to male or White counterparts, **Black women regardless of socioeconomic status had the highest levels of allostatic load** (Geronimus).

RJ centers on the act that the human being that created harm did. RJ lasers in on the harm and the impact of harm caused to other human beings and the community. It is the act that is hoped to never occur again, and it is the human that will be held accountable to community by being an active participant in making the wrong right. **In short, we banish the act of harm and help**

those who created the harm see the hurt they caused while they work to fix the harm.

"Everyone belongs in a circle. And the circle is always directed towards healing from the harm of disconnection." (Pranis)

There is significant preparation work that takes place before bringing conflicting parties together for RJ practices. No one is ever thrown away or deemed monster, predator or unworthy of sharing their story before corrective action occurs. RJ does not make excuses for the actions people who created harm did. **Nor does RJ expect forgiveness from the person/people that were harmed.** RJ does expect that conditions will be set for respectful conversation and decision-making of all parties involved to come up with a solution to the harm. Preparation is honestly the most important part of the restorative process.

Skilled restorative practitioners are gifted at holding brave space so that each person involved is empowered to speak openly about the event of harm and its impact on their lives (Long). Accountability comes when all those involved have a stake in the outcome. It is the acts of empowerment and respect for each human present in the process that promotes collaborative repair.

These acts also promote (health) equity by including people who are often unheard or unseen by the system. This advances solutions and healing by building community and trust (Long).

RJ is intentional about building capacity to convene groups in a respectful environment (e.g., circles, conferences) which leads to dialogue, healing, accountability and problem solving amongst all those affected by an incident (Long). It is this uniqueness of RJ's reparative techniques that deepens trust, opens individuals to share perspectives, and facilitates collective decisions on the next steps (Long).

Soon, we will take a look at real life examples of Restorative Justice in practice for health crises inside and outside of the United States. It is only right that we understand the full context of the origins of restorative justice. These practices began with the rise of societies and civilizations. It's hard to say exactly when it, RJ, started. It is very clear that communal boundaries, rules or suggestions of ways to live together came about 12,000-40,000 years ago. My dear, I was not there when it popped off. Nor, can I say that the recordkeeping from that era translates very well.

What I do know is that Indigenous people are all over this world. They are the settlers of land as far as records

go back. There are 5,000 distinct Indigenous communities spread across 90 countries in the world. Collectively,
there are 476 million people that identify as Indigenous.
And we know that since the beginning of time, communities have used restorative practices to keep the
peace in the land (Davis) and address problems through
knowledge sharing (YassieCJ).

There are several modern-day teachers of Restorative
Justice that have created a foundation of which most
RJ practitioners work from. Since the 1980s, Chief
Justice Robert Yazzie has publicly taught that "where
there is hurt, there must be healing" referencing the
Navajo Nation's Restorative Practices. The intention has
been to bring balance back to the community to restore
peace after disruption. Prompted by the hurt of mass
incarceration of Indigenous people, members of the
First Nations in Canada began working and teaching
outside of the Indigenous community to halt the modern-day genocide (Restorative). Partnerships amongst
Indigenous and Non-Indigenous Allies have made
tremendous impact around the world within the criminal
justice, juvenile justice, and schools' systems. Indigenous Tlingit Leaders Mark Wedge and Harold Gatensby
and Canadian Chief Justice Barry Stuart teach that they
*"pass this (RJ/Peacekeeping) on to everyone as a gift
to use to promote healthy communities"* (CEL). Around

this same time, the Afrocentric Restorative Justice framework was shared by Professor and Chair of the Department of Criminal Justice and Social Work Morris Jenkins.

Professor Jenkins notes that the foundation of restorative practices is "just law" in an effort to "make things whole" and "make the community whole" (Davis, Jenkins). Dr. Jenkins highlights the traditional ways of living and peace keeping that the people of the Gullah Island have held with them since before being enslaved and transported to the United States (Jenkins). **The common thread among all the listed communities seems to be respect for the humanity of each person involved, respectful dialogue to problem-solve and restore peace and build trust.**

Current day, Restorative Justice continues to be used in Indigenous communities and is being applied in a variety of situations (Davis, Karp). You can see RJ in action in the judicial courts (Mirsky), nonprofits, tenuous communities, K-12 education and recently graduate communities (Davis, Karp, AAMC, Behel). I think the world saw one of the greatest examples of restorative practices with the fall of apartheid in South Africa. The Truth and Reconciliation Commission (TRC) implemented

RJ practices after the atrocities of apartheid to create collaborative law and establish respect for all people under the South African flag.

Restorative Practices are even making their way to healthcare (Long, AAMC, Behel, Wailing, NHS, Health-careCAN). Abroad, New Zealand, Canada and the UK are noted for implementing large scale RJ programs to understand the needs of vulnerable patients and with those patients create solutions to advance the quality and compassion of healthcare (Long). Within the U.S., organizations such as radical Health (Bronx, NY) are bridging "the gap between systemically marginalized communities and the medical system" by empowering patients with information and advocacy on their terms.

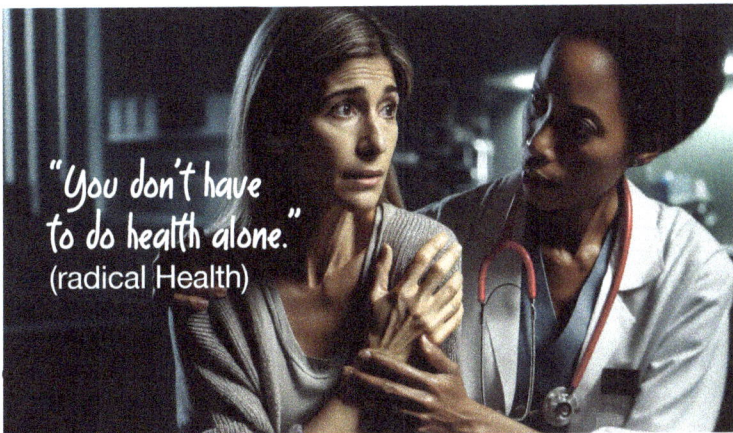

"You don't have to do health alone."
(radical Health)

It is in the absence of dialogue that fear, panic, and angst go unchecked and lead to more harm. As an example, in real life we saw the absence of dialogue lead to mob attacks and mass poisonings that occurred during the early days of the COVID-19 Pandemic (Coleman). Even large organizations, such as the Association of American Medical Colleges (AAMC), are training providers and educators to shift the response to harm and foster community and healing with Restorative Justice practices.

In practice, RJ respectfully brings together people that have a shared stake in a situation to share insights and problem-solve after a traumatic situation. "A central practice of restorative justice is the collaborative decision-making process that includes harmed parties, people who have caused harm, and others who are seeking active accountability" (Darling). These coming together events are strictly voluntary. The framework of RJ promotes peace and understanding by removing the social distance between people by highlighting our interconnectedness (Pranis). These are the actions that correct unjust policies and promote healing.

RJ Facilitators guide all concerned parties to consider and address the root causes that create the conditions for such vile acts of harm to occur. **When stakeholders**

drill down, it is often systemic (large scale policies) inequities and social injustices that fertilize the hurt. Collaborative plans to respond to the harm often target the conditions and root causes of harm.

My hope for marginalized communities is to engage with Restorative Justice to advance productive partnerships amongst patient, provider and healthcare systems. Restorative justice can be applied in several different ways or tiers to address harm. Starting at the bottom or level 0, there is a call to **create readiness** within a community. It is at this foundational point that RJ is introduced to people, making them aware of restorative justice and the impact of RJ (AAMC).

The next level is often for **relationship building amongst people in a shared community.** This is where trust begins, by opening the door to communication amongst various people. Often restorative justice practices are geared towards **repairing harm and rebuilding trust** after misconduct or a traumatic event (Karp). Lastly, Restorative Justice has been helpful in **providing supportive accountability** towards members that have been apart from the community due to medical illness, incarceration, suspension, etc. (Karp). Experienced RJ Facilitators are skillful at determining which tier of RJ to implement for each situation. It is essential that each stage should be facilitated by a competent and experienced RJ facilitator (Long). **The goal is not to create harm in an attempt to facilitate problem-solving to address a hurt.**

At the heart of restorative justice, no one is to be thrown away! People are not one dimensional. No one is only their worst decision or indefinitely stuck in purgatory from their worst action. "Everyone belongs in a circle. And the circle is always directed towards healing from the harm of disconnection" (Pranis). **With guided reflection and respectful communication, new ways of navigating life can be co-created** (Kaba). The goal of RJ "is not to assign blame to individual providers or organizations" for past harms. Instead, all people with a stake in a situation discuss patterns of harms and exclusion in the affected communities. This helps contextualize limitations of current policies and practices and shapes healthier future policy. "These collaborative processes build bridges of trust between communities, patients, and providers by allowing each group to understand how others have been impacted by the healthcare crisis. The end result is a win-win for equity and health justice in the serviced community" (Long).

Within healthcare, there is a lot of room for restorative justice practices. History has shown over and over again that "under resourcing, misinforming, and segregating access to care and training for Black, Indigenous, People of Color (BIPOC)/Latinx communities" is a very common (Long), almost routine phenomenon.

Disenfranchising healthcare recipients by maintaining barriers to quality healthcare "consistently correlate to higher disease burden, death and mental distress amongst BIPOC/Latinx communities (Long)." **Including the voices of those who receive medical care disrupts this phenomenon of hurt/harm.** Inclusion of vulnerable voices breaks "centuries-long patterns of excluding marginalized communities from medical decision-making" (Long). Such inclusion can actually protect vulnerable communities by eliminating the threat of harm and build protective measures for these communities to thrive (Long). To have maximum benefit from RJ practices, it is important that patients and providers speak the same language and have a similar context for the events that lead up to the harm. **This is where community building begins by sharing context without blame.** The uninterrupted sharing of such experiences brings awareness to the embodied experiences of marginalized people. Oftentimes marginalized communities are bringing their personal and communal trauma to medical encounters.

Therapist and Healer Resmaa Menakem says, "Trauma in a person, decontextualized over time, looks like personality. Trauma in a family, decontextualized over time, looks like family traits. Trauma in a people, decontextualized over time, looks like culture! (Fragoso).

There is an opportunity for healthcare to truly be part of the solution of healing from toxic stress and othering with restorative practices. This is an achievable goal with institutional buy-in. RJ plants the seed of awareness which allows healing outcomes to follow.

There are opportunities for restorative justice to be utilized to strengthen community and to break down the silos between patients and caregivers. RJ implemented at the beginning of the relationship before the harm has occurred leads to success for all parties involved. Opportunities are created for all parties to share authentically and to achieve common goals for great health. RJ is truly a chance to get to know our neighbors and understand their needs. Fania Davis, JD, PhD, shares that when RJ becomes official policy, it "proactively strengthens community." This makes space for each person to accept responsibly for their part in an event which can repair harm.

When Restorative Practices are implemented through-out an organization. It is paramount that all parties engaging in the process understand the origins of these practices. When done with high fidelity, organizations should engage with local Indigenous Communities, particularly the Elders, to partner and benefit from the organization's use of Restorative Practices.

When we look outside of the United States, Restorative Justice has been used on a very large scale to address medical harm and trauma. In 2017, our neighbors to the north in Canada respectfully engaged in Indigenous Communities in creating the "Wise Practices." This is an example of national level Restorative Practices that addressed healthcare disparities and inequities of mar-ginalized communities. Partnerships were developed between First Nations communities, Traditional Healers, healthcare organizations, and medical learners "to ensure inclusion of traditional healing in the primary care models in ways that are respectful, responsive" (IW) and patient empowering. Explicit attention was paid to the impact of racism's impact on health and wellness. "Experiences of racism have been reported in multiple Indigenous survey studies, across a variety of geograph-ic settings" (HealthcareCAN).

One Canadian study, for example, "found that Indigenous patients strategized about how to manage racism
before presenting in a hospital emergency department,
and also worried that their health concerns would be
dismissed because of assumptions made about them
by health providers" (HealthcareCAN).

The Wise Practices report gave concrete steps to help
HealthcareCAN organizations implement anti-racist
practices which include: "Provide anti-racism and cultural safety education to all members of the organization; develop and implement safe processes for both
employees and clients to debrief racist or culturally
unsafe experiences in the organization; develop and
implement processes to document these instances
and track progress" (HealthcareCAN). "When health
care providers adopt a trauma-informed approach, they
consider a person's reactions (such as treatment refusal
or mistrust) as a possible result of previous experience
or injury, rather than just as sickness or bad behaviour"
(HealthcareCAN). Such practices get phenomenal
results. In 2013, the Indigenous Health Authority
launched a "Diabetes & My Nation" program in British
Columbia (Dawson). The community co-created diabetes care for their members and designed lifestyle and
physical activity programs on the basis of tailored cultural
traditions. The diabetes outcomes were better in this

community than in communities with programs led by primary care. In 2023, $8.2 billion and directive control allocated to First Nations Health Authority in Canada by the government. "This renewal is about improving delivery and meeting the unique health needs of First Nations communities with things like more community-based approaches to health care, recognition of the intergenerational trauma that impacts well-being in your communities," Prime Minister Trudeau (Torre). "The key was a shared solution design and culturally enriched practices" (Liu).

In 2017, the National Health Services (NHS) in the UK implemented restorative practices in the duty of candor campaign. There was a very structured, respectful way medical errors and high-risk events were disclosed to patients and family members and collaboratively practices were changed to reduce harms other people.

In 2019, the New Zealand Government's Ministry of Health used restorative practices to understand the psychological and physical harm of botched surgical mesh repairs for hernia cost. In a very respectful way, the health ministry identified practices that alienated patients and weakened the culture of safety within healthcare. The results of this collaboration reduced future physical and moral injury to both patient and healthcare providers.

Look around, there's an abundance of opportunities to apply these practices locally. The pandemic and every natural disaster (e.g., winter storm, earthquake, torna-do) presents an opportunity to grow together. RJ can foster communication to acknowledge the pain and hurt of survivors, shore up practices to reduce future harms, and establish trust for future disaster scenarios. **It's very important that the people at the epicenter of harmful events are included in policy creation.** Those at the greatest margins are the most vulnerable. Marginalized communities are often disenfranchised and not empowered during good times. Times of crisis only exacerbates the conditions for these communities (EJI).

The next level of restorative practices center around not throwing anyone away and engaging everyone involved to create accountability for harmful actions. Even after people have been separated from their communities by incarceration, death, performance review, etc., **high quality restorative practices have leveled the playing field to help communities regroup and move forward in the healthiest way possible.** RJ illuminates the weight of uncertainty and the depths of disappointment from an untoward event.

In its finest application, restorative justice has been utilized to bring together murderers and the family that they hurt. These gatherings do not occur overnight. They do occur after lots of reflection and insight from all parties involved. The collective results of RJ consistently show a reduction in future harmful events. Even more, the affected communities often feel safer and more empowered because there's been an established agreement of how to engage the community. There is an explicit understanding of all involved what appropriate plans and actions will occur if the agreement is not adhered to or is broken. The applications of RJ are as expansive as people can imagine.

The road ahead will be determined by three key things coming together in a respectful way. The gift that results from these elements coming together can be curated in such a way that future generations can benefit from the collective efforts. It will require brave reflective work within and between individuals, small groups of marginalized communities, and then collectively. **Every step of the way will bring moments of discomfort, AND this is okay.** It is the brave space that RJ holds which allows the discomfort to be managed and growth can occur from there (Long).

The individual work is the internal prep work that clarifies individual needs and reflects on unjust or harmful events. **This space clarifies what would make each stakeholder seen and/or honor the memory of those loved ones lost along the way.** As a living human being, each patient and their supporters are worthy of respect and high-quality care. It is important that each stakeholder defines what respect in healthcare would look like.

Next, it is important to come together in small groups with similar people who have experienced such harms. The power in this step is the individual healing of loneliness and isolation that occur when people realize they are not alone. Lifting the veil of embarrassment and shame from intimate medical procedures going awry is life changing. It is when the small groups with common interests (e.g., disability, English as Second Language) come together that patterns of harm can start to be identified (Long). Stakeholders are prepped during this stage to identify values and hopes for future improvements. The patterns of harm and values identified become the compass for the new policy creation. **Stakeholders, not facilitators, are seen as experts in this process because they have the insight of lived experience.** This unleashes the power of RJ, the ability to innovate creative solutions from dark times.

The circle grows larger during the next phase of RJ. The marginalized communities are respectfully introduced to one another in a collective effort for structural change and next steps creation (Long). This is the point when all involved in policy creation come together for information gathering and the act of respectful dialogue with one another. **This only happens with preparation, respectful facilitation, and a willingness for accountability.** The gifts that are created during this phase are the efforts that will reduce harmful events for future patients. These gifts are drafted into policies that clearly identify process flow or how operations are supposed to run in a very transparent way. Everyone gets on the same page here. There is one pivotal component that must not be overlooked. Once the collective is together, it is important that the question of: Who's not in the room with us? is addressed. Lasting community can only be built when all parties are brave and acknowledge who may be missing from the room (or conversation) and acknowledge that blind spots are present. **Those blind spots are often the key which limits the potential of creative solutions. It truly is when diversity of thought sits around the table together that innovation can occur.** It's the acts of being brave and acknowledging that there are things we may not know or experience differently that parties involved feel safe enough (psychological safety) to speak candidly without fear of being hurt again.

The practice of listening without expressing judgement is the secret that makes restorative justice practices magical. It must be explicitly stated that "safe" spaces are not the goal, rather brave space is the goal. What makes one person feel safe may not necessarily make another feel safe. For example, ten guns on the table in the middle of the room may make some feel very secure. For other people, those ten guns on the table can provoke fear and possibly terror.

Once the collective has been assembled, all stakeholders must create a system of accountability that seems just. This creates a level of transparency and reduces the anxiety of what if, what if the act occurs again. Even folks that have created harm are empowered not to recreate the harm because they have a full understanding of the impact of their act and are engaged in being part of the solution. As the streets say: the code must be respected. The scholars have seen proof of this concept. Repeat harm creation (Wailing) and recidivism (Davis) are reduced from thoughtful restorative practices. **It is through collective action that innovation and long-lasting solutions are developed and hold weight.** There is magic in the acknowledgment of the worth of each stakeholder regardless of title or social stature. Transformative change truly occurs when lived experience is held in equal esteem as statistical data.

By including all stakeholders at the start of the process, transparency is created around the entire process. As the stakeholders get further and further away from the initial days of policy creation, the written action plan of accountability will serve as a north star to keep all parties on track and honest about the intention of efforts. **These actions empower marginalized communities, expand the knowledge base of scholars, and reduce the mismatch between policy and practice in healthcare delivery.** Once the action plans have been created, it is of great importance to make the information publicly available to all who engage with the healthcare system.

Fancy technology is not necessary to start on the road to trust building and collaborative solution creation through RJ. Starting with the resources at hand and a genuine concern to partner in a long-lasting relationship with the harmed community is key. As this process requires significant intentionality, it is helpful to have trained Restorative Justice Facilitators guide the process from the individual to the collective acts. The facilitators help all parties thrive after harm and not just get over the hurt (Boyes-Watson).

When the facilitation has been done well with the

intention of collective input, the results are always mind-blowing. Those who have lived with the pain of hurt from medical injustice and those who know they have blood on their hands, can find a way forward together. The New Zealand patients and medical providers had a deeper understanding of each other's pressures and impacts to life from botched surgical procedures. Collectively, new standards for medical practices, certification for performing such practices and support for patient follow-up were established. **In short, RJ done well can: promote collaborative repair (of relationships) for all involved (Davis), promotes health equity through inclusion while building community and provider trust, and mitigate risk** (the chance that bad things will continue to happen) (Long). Often the first level of healing encompasses patients and providers who have caused harm. As the Honorable Chief Justice Yazzie said, "But the relatives would also feel relief, and those who are also interested in the process would feel the same way. So in the end, there's healing at different levels" (Mirsky). Ultimately, peace, healing and understanding are achieved for the entire community and future generations. Promotion of health equity must not occur in isolation. The historical context of community care and trauma must be accounted for. Otherwise, there will be a skewed version of the present social situation of how all parties got to this point.

The goal is not to reproduce systems of oppression (Davis, SAEM). Similarly, healthcare interventions should not be given unlimited authority, the factual limitations of medical devices and procedures should be acknowledged (SAEM). Transparency will lighten the load of burden that all involved experience, including the untold second casualties. Many frontline healthcare workers suffer from increased risk of infection, death, and mental health crisis from secondarily being exposed to inequitable systems (Long). "RJ offers a framework by which community and clinical stakeholders can collaborate" to create solutions that "address the needs of those affected," reduce the chance that such a wrong will ever happen again (CRJ), and reduce the burden of the moral injury everyone involved carries. RJ processes build trust by allowing people to increase understanding through communication. These are some of the steps that will make health inequities a memory of the past and build hope for a brighter, healthier future.

In closing, Dr. Long wants you to know that you and those you love are worthy of respectful, competent care. You are powerful enough to hold the healthcare system accountable and reap the benefits of high-quality care, no matter the zip code you happen to be in during a healthcare encounter.

Engaging with the healthcare
system or receiving healthcare is like being
the baton in a relay race. At any point during
an exchange, things can go sideways leading
to a tremendous setback or loss.
Teamwork with everyone engaged
in the system makes it likely
that there will be fewer
baton drops/errors/hurts.

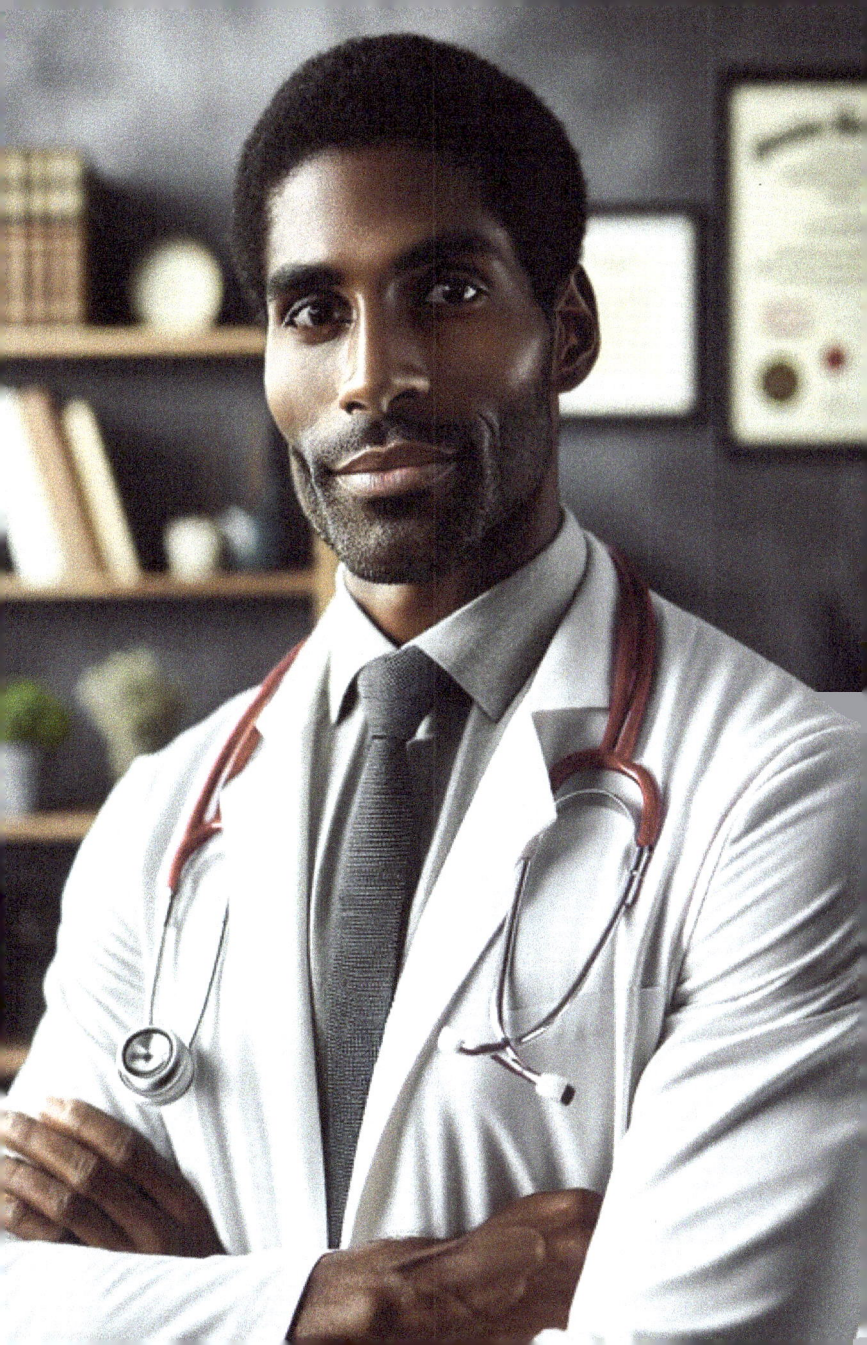

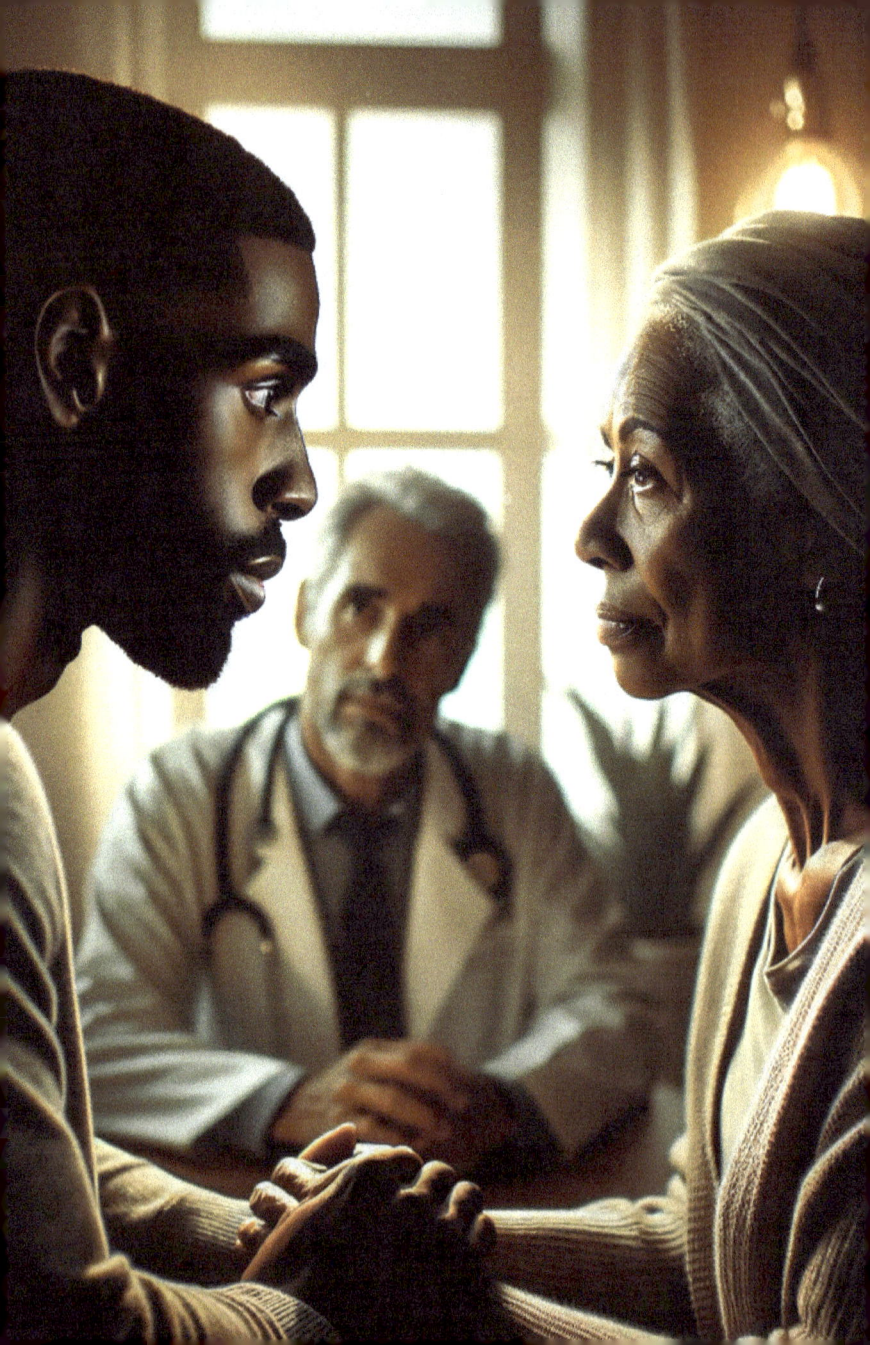

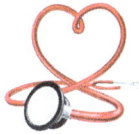

Chapter 13

Helpful Practices When Engaging the Healthcare System

• **Take a deep breath** to help clear your thinking and release some of the tension in your body. Do this just before you enter into the healthcare facility **and again** shortly after being checked-in for service.

• Let someone close to you (e.g., confidant, homie, partner) know that you are going to the hospital to seek care. Even better if they can accompany you.

• If you have to attend the healthcare facility alone, consider taking a cell phone and charger with you. This way when doctors and providers come in and explain your care, you can call your ace to have a second pair of ears to hear the information as well. Many times, we only hear bits and pieces of information when we are scared and/or in pain. Introduce your ace to the provider, just as though they were physically in the room with you.

• If you live with a disability, as 1 in 4 people in the United States (CDC D), know that **you have the right** to full and equal access to healthcare. Healthcare facilities are required to make reasonable accommodation to provide patients with disabilities with equitable care (ADANN). For example, the ADA (Americans with Disabilities Act) is the federal civil rights law that gives people who are deaf and hard of hearing the right to effective communication in healthcare settings at no cost. Thus, interpreters and modifications to visitation policies are permissible to allow the person with the disability to benefit to the fullest extent of healthcare services (ADANN Aux).

• If English is not your native language or you have limited English proficiency, ask for a native language interpreter. By federal law and executive order, an interpreter (verbal or sign language) should be provided at no extra expense to you (USDJ).

• If you ever get in a **situation where you feel you haven't been heard,** you can ask for a patient care advocate, patient liaison or patient navigator to help you work your way to trusted answers from the system. These specialists can help you in communicating with your healthcare team.

• If you feel tension communicating why you showed up at this moment, take a moment to be vulnerable to your healthcare provider. Say what your fear is about this current situation and what responsibilities you have. For example, say "I am scared/fearful that this headache is a stroke, and I need to provide for my children and grandkids."

• **Let's practice:** If a doctor, nurse, or tech says something that is unclear or uncomfortable, take a deep breath. Then say, "I know there is a lot going on in the department right now. I just think it would be helpful if I knew this wasn't cancer or stroke, miscarriage, etc. How do you know for certain that this is not cancer or stroke, miscarriage? I want to be alive for my family." This practice will make the situation less hostile and will humanize the person in front of the healthcare provider.

• ** <u>It is never okay to verbally or physically abuse medical staff/providers</u>. Additionally, violence against healthcare providers is scary, disruptive, and lessens the quality of care other patients receive in that facility. There is a push to immediately use teams of people to de-escalate volatile situations. In circumstances that are beyond the scope of de-escalation, law enforcement engagement and felony charges can result (Boyle P). There are motions underway to make such acts federal felonies (Muoio).

The intent is not to excuse unprofessional or subpar healthcare worker behavior. Rather it is to understand that during crisis and excessive stress, healthcare workers are people who struggle as well. Many take home the weight of many patients' problems with them at the end of the day. Our profession has a dirty secret of healthcare worker casualties. Healthcare workers suffer from increased risk of infection, death, and mental health crisis from being exposed to such trauma (Long). Many healthcare workers carry this moral trauma with them for life.

For example, providers on the frontlines from emergency department, intensive care, and infectious disease units had risks for anxiety, depression and suicide from caring for COVID-19 patients and the constraints of operating during a prolonged crisis state (Long). At times of excessive stress, many folks stop thinking with their rational mind and default to learned patterns. Many folks call these implicit biases, thereby limiting the stressed person's ability to make the best judgement in this current situation (Fragoso, Davis).

Dr. Ruby J. Long

In the ideal world, all conditions would be right to allow patients to receive "accurate, easily understood information to help them make informed decisions about their health plans, professionals and facilities" (OPM). Additionally, patients would truly feel and know that all communications and records about care will be treated as confidential to the extent permitted by law (NIH).

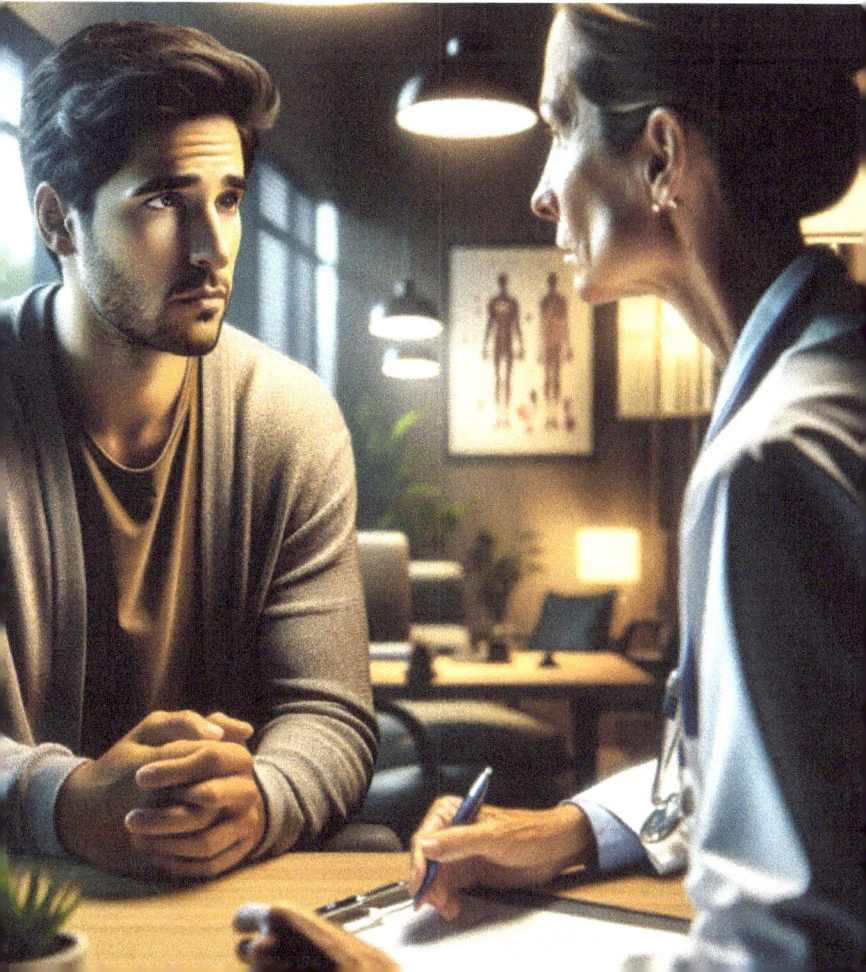

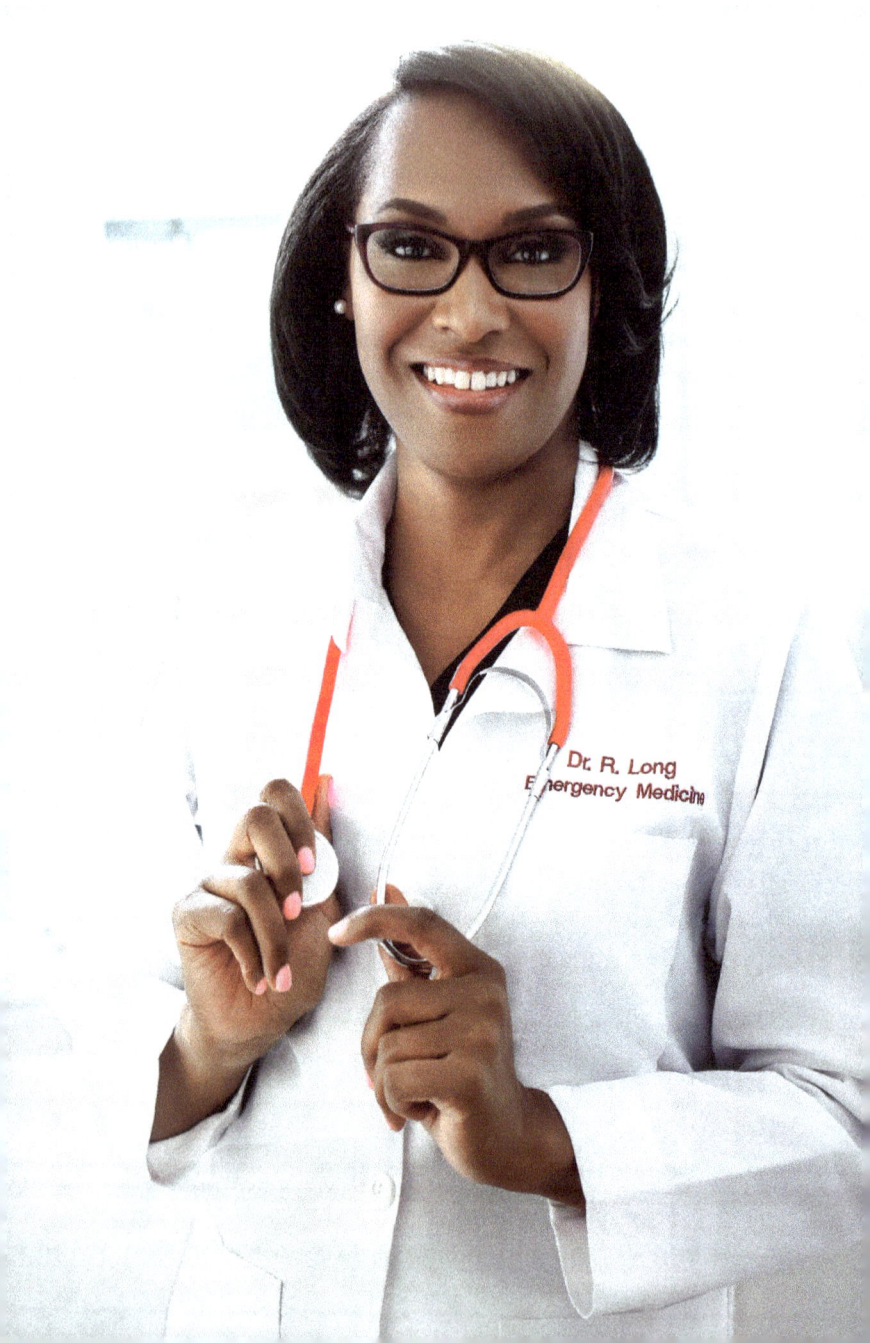

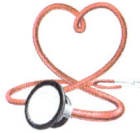

Chapter 14

Dr. Ruby J. Long's Love Letter of Gratitude to Patients

Compassionate Letter

As a **Board-Certified Emergency Physician** who has worked in urban, rural, and academic medical center sites, my heart was forever ripped open by the COVID pandemic. I know trauma firsthand. It's what I trained so long for. Car accidents, interpersonal violence (guns, knives, fists/feet against another person) and industrial accidents required a high level of preparation to give those harmed the best chance at survival. Thus, when COVID came and began to terrorize communities, I knew exactly what I was looking at: the start of generational trauma.

We, the public, often think of COVID in isolation. We think: COVID has taken XYZ from me, my routine, my family. In actuality COVID has a very wide reach. COVID took over a million of lives in the U.S. and almost 7 million human lives around the world (WHO D). Unfortunately, no matter how lonely we feel, we are not a planet of ones. We are a planet of communities. Each person counted in the loss from COVID was connected somehow. They were the bread earners, doing the honorable jobs for their families (e.g., sweeping floors, driving buses, stocking shelves). They were keeping society going.

Our Lost Loves were the primary caregivers for young children and aging elders. They were people who had potential for innovation, love and laughter. So, when I really think of the impact of COVID, I can see families being ripped from their homes, children without the person who looked out for them, elders transitioning from this life alone, and all the love and laughter we as a society will miss out on. This generation will take the scars of COVID with us. The hope is that it is not in vain as the ripples of the lost ones flow out.

I look forward to the day when people can engage healthcare services and not feel that they are making a choice between a bad decision and a really fucked up decision.

I wrote this book to let patients know they are loved and they matter. So many times, when patients and their families of love show up on the worst day of their lives, they grace me with gifts. I want to be very clear and say **thank you** for sharing the most vulnerable moments of your life with me. Thank you for giving me a kind word when hope seems lost. These actions of unselfishness fill me up with energy. They help me speak up and speak out when I know the healthcare system can do better. Thank you for seeing me and oftentimes sharing your pride that I get to care for you.

Thank you for giving me grace when I have been rushed or distracted. Thank you for partnering with me and starting this trust walk to make healthcare better. Your compassion during times of trials restores my soul. It means everything to see such acts of kindness and gratitude during these dark days.

Shout out to my I-65 fam. I've driven that highway from end to end thinking of your stories. Because of your sacrifices and dreams, I'm grateful that I could have better opportunities. Thank you, too, for being a village that raised and loved me and DID NOT SMASH MY DREAMS. Thank you to my Ezell and Long Elders who held infinite wisdom and hope that their children could create hope for the future.

It is my hope that collectively patients/advocates/ providers can bring healing back to healthcare. My goal was to empower patients/patient advocates with knowledge of their worth as humans and worthiness of respectful quality healthcare. I will continue the work of encouraging health systems to review their application of policies, the implicit biases of their team members, and the power of the social systems they represent. In closing, to all those who are touched by this book, **my wish is that you are heard the first time you and your loves show up for healthcare.** I look forward to the day when the experts with the lived experience of being part of a marginalized community are truly listened to and not spoken over. The act of embracing truthful storytelling to shape policy and practices will change the world for the benefit of all of humanity. I truly see restorative justice as a systemic answer for hope. Wrapping you all in love.

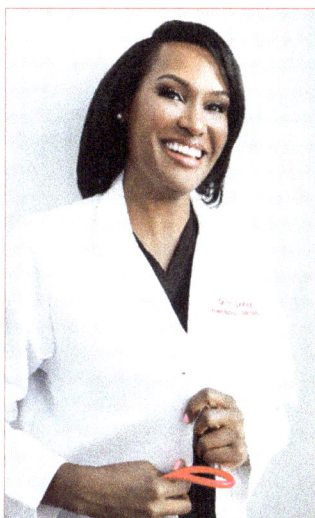

Earnestly,

Dr. Ruby J. Long

Dr. Ruby J. Long

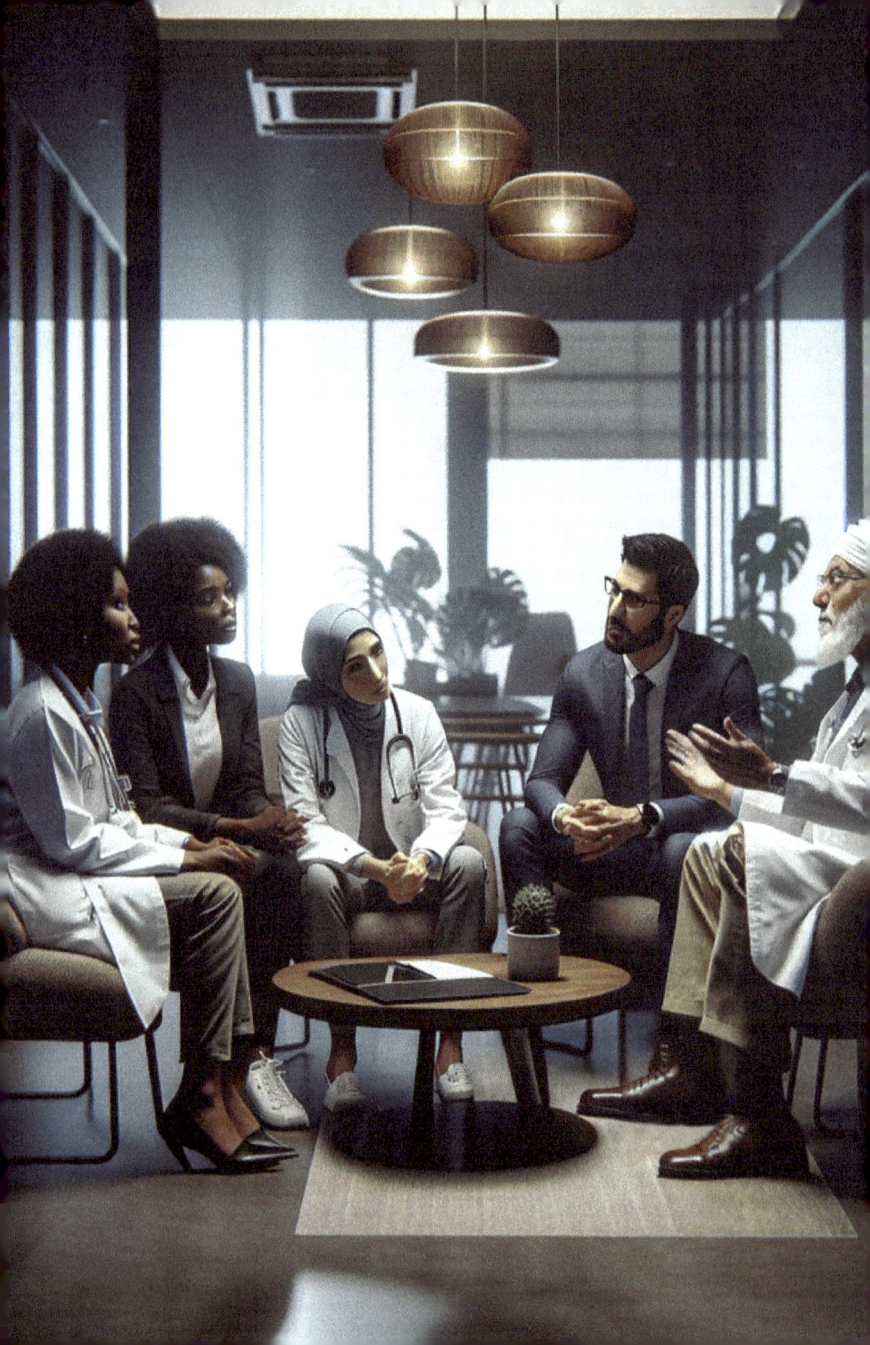

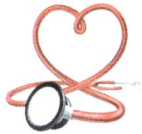

Chapter 15

Dr. Ruby J. Long's Heart-to-Heart Letter to Other Providers

Dear Health Care Workers, I commend you for reading this book and being an active partner with patients. I'm sure many of you are familiar with what I am about to write. However, I want to make the nebulous explicit, as this is not often done in our training. At the heart of the matter, patients want to be seen!

Patients also want to be seen as human beings worthy of dignity and respect. Patients yearn to be seen for their unique personalities and layers of their lives.

Our first moments with patients require our greatest attention. It is in these first moments that patients give or withhold their trust in us as healers. It is of the greatest importance that when you enter the room of a patient, that patient in front of you becomes your biggest priority.

Your personal matters (e.g., fights with partners, compensation, work hours, stock portfolio, etc.) must fall into the background. This requires a moment of self-preparation to be truly present as you enter the treatment space. You must do a check-in with yourself to figure out how to ground yourself and be present for the patient encounter.

Once you are truly present, then enter the patient's treatment space. Remember, the patients came for healing or the hope to maintain good health. As you enter the healing space, your pace, the cadence of your voice, eye contact, and introductions or lack thereof are being noted. Introductions are key. Please let patients know who you are as you enter the space. You might even say, Hello or "I'm glad to care for you today."

Then proceed to ask the patient their name or who they are. This can be a slippery slope. Elders are often attached to titles (Mr., Mrs., Ms., Dr.), as many see them as a sign of respect and honor. This generation of folks have often been looked over by those in power. This is extremely true for women and racial/ethnic marginalized communities that had to engage the U.S. Supreme Court for human rights protections. More youthful patients may take greater pride in not being labeled with honorifics. This often applies to non-binary/gender diverse people.

Many in the LGBTQ+ community have had gender labels weaponized against them intentionally to harm or diminish their self-worth. It is best not to make assumptions about a patient's gender. It might be best to just ask the patient what their name is and how they identify, or what do they prefer that you call them.

If people feel disrespected or unseen in the first moments of the encounter, they may not engage in the recommended care plan or withhold information that could be lifesaving (e.g., not disclosing organs they were born with such as breasts or penis, then missing the opportunity for preventative cancer screening).

During the interview and examination, really listen

to what the patient and/or their family's report. Acknowledge their concerns and provide those seeking care with tools to empower themselves with the best evidence-based therapies available. Make it clear that the patient is in control to choose the path of care they feel most in alignment with and will be supported in their efforts. At the close of the encounter, consider asking the patient and their family of choice, "Is there anything else you have a concern about?" You even might share a moment of gratitude with the patient for letting you care for them.

Please tap into that desire to truly help others that originally piqued your interest in healthcare. Patients are counting on it. Honestly, if the glimmer is gone and the new normal has become power over others or just a paycheck, please do reflect on what profession could bring you joy. It is the joy that people see in your work that makes them reflect back joyously to you.

With love, compassion and gratitude for your service,

Dr. Ruby J. Long

Dr. Ruby J. Long

If you get tired, learn to rest, not quit.
— Banksy

_____

_____

_____

_____

_____

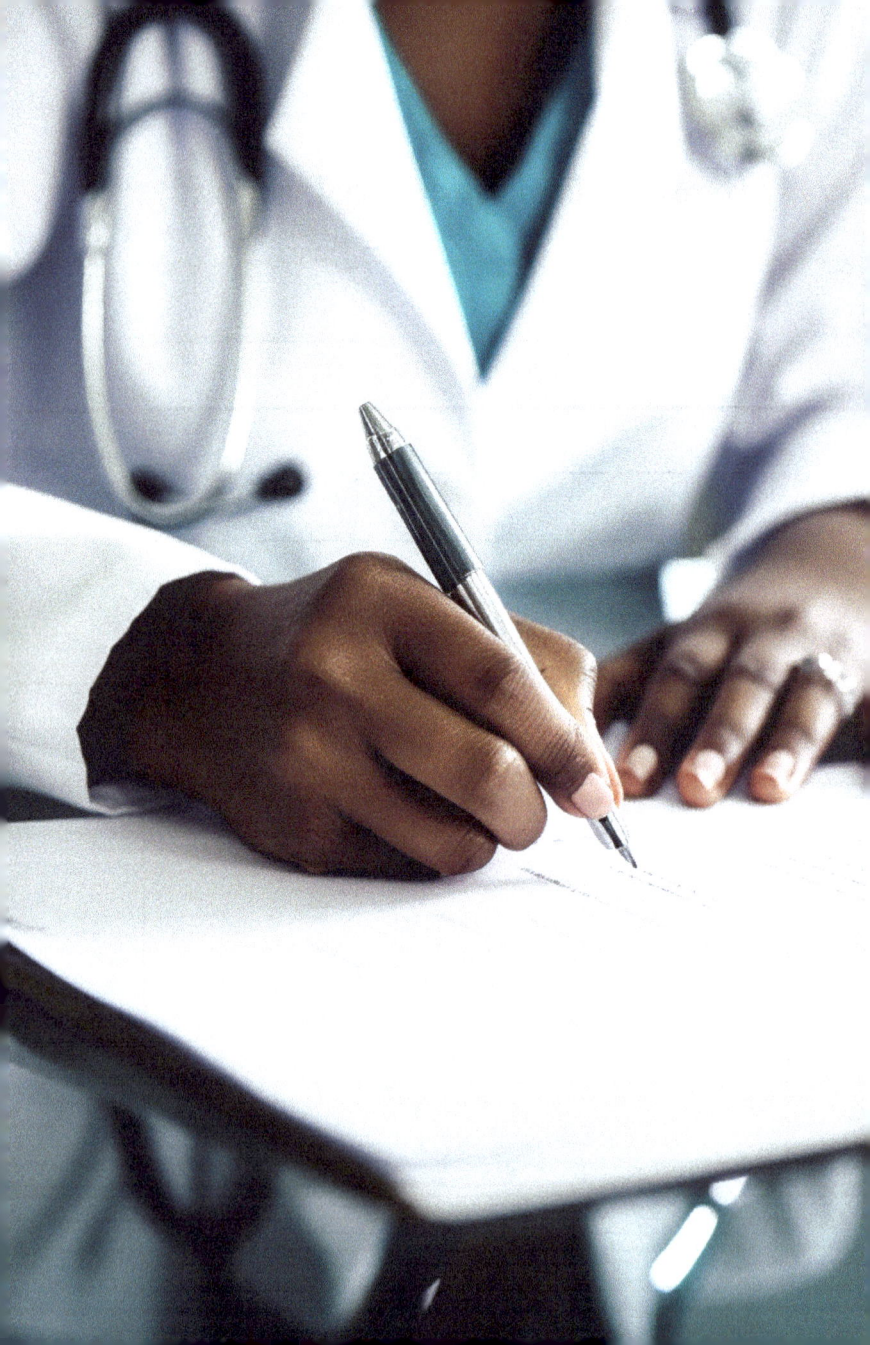

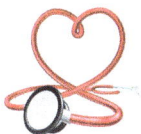

Chapter 16

Patient Health History

- Name

- Allergies

- Medical Conditions

- Surgeries

- Primary Care Doctor/Provider

- Specialty Doctor/Provider
  (Cardiologist, Neurologist, OB/Gyn)

- In Case of Emergency **(ICE)** Contact: (Name)
  (Phone Number)

Patient Wishes

These are not legally binding documents, just insight to your wishes. Please engage your lawyer or your primary healthcare provider to establish formal advance directives.

If I, _____ (insert your name), am unable to speak for myself during a catastrophic, life threatening SHORT-TERM medical event, I _____ (fill in your wish here, e.g., I do not or I do) want to have life sustaining interventions such as life support: chest compressions (e.g., CPR), intubation (e.g. airway breathing tube) and mechanical ventilation (e.g. machine that internally breaths for me).

_____
Patient Signature

_____
Date

These are not legally binding documents, just insight to your wishes. Please engage your lawyer or your primary healthcare provider to establish formal advance directives.

If I, _____ (insert your name), am unable to speak for myself during a catastrophic, life threatening LONG-TERM / PRO-LONGED medical event greater than one month, I _____ (fill in your wish here e.g. I do not or I do) want to have life sustaining interventions such as life support: chest compressions (e.g., CPR), intubation (e.g., airway breathing tube) and mechanical ventilation (e.g., machine that internally breaths for me).

_____

Patient Signature

_____

Date

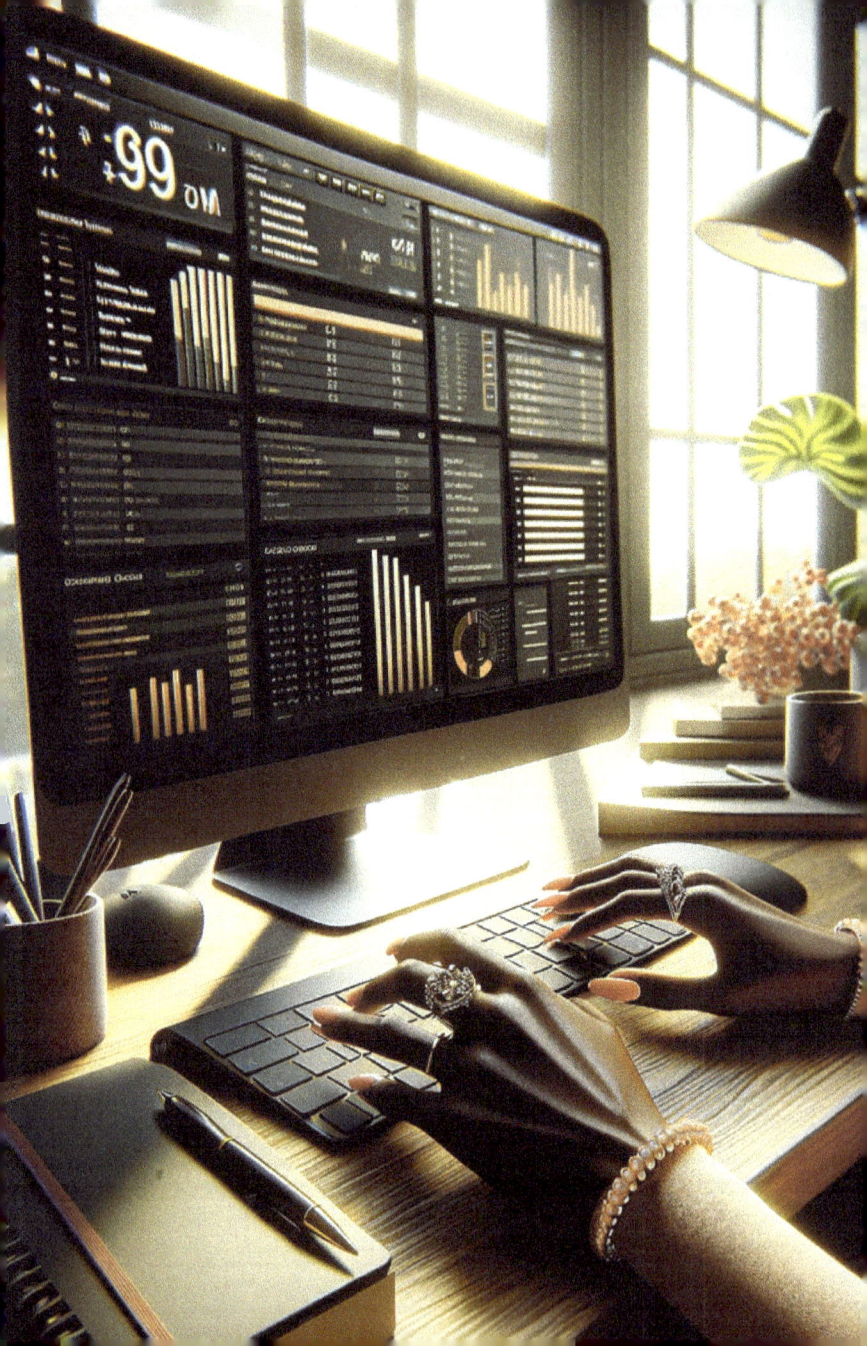

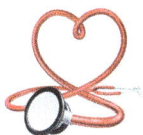

Chapter 17

Resources

Pearls for Health

Resources

Emergencies

Threat to life or limb (e.g. stroke, heart attack, complicated childbirth, etc.)

• Call 9-1-1, Llame 9-1-1

Overdose

Give naloxone/Narcan© and call EMS if somone has blue lips and not breathing well. Si los labios azules y ellos no respira bien.

• Call 9-1-1, Llame 9-1-1
(Substance use help – SAMHSA)

Suicide

Help is always available. If you have thoughts of hurting yourself:

• **Call 988** for assistance.

• Para ayuda en español, **llame al 988**.

Violence: Lover

Love is not being controlled or hit.

• National Domestic Violence Hotline **(800) 799-SAFE (7233)** or text **88788**.

• TTY for the hearing-impaired at (800) 787-3224.

Violence: Gendered

Love is not being controlled or hit.

• Rape Abuse & Incest National Network (RAINN) Hotline **(800) 656-HOPE (4673)**.

Violence: Elderly

"If you have been the victim of abuse, exploitation, or neglect, you are not alone" (HHS).

• Eldercare Locator help line **1-800-677-1116**.

• SAGE's National LGBT Elder Hotline **877-360-LGBT**.

Violence: Children

Children deserve to live to their full potential without threat of abuse or neglect.

• **Childhelp® National Child Abuse Hotline (800)-4-A-CHILD (1-800-422-4453).**

Violence: Guns/Firearms

BE SMART

Secure all guns in your homes and vehicles

Model responsible behavior around guns

Ask about unsecured guns in other homes

Recognize the role of guns in suicide

Tell your peers to Be SMART

• **BeSMARTforKids.org**
For tips or to get involved, text SMART to 644-33.

• **Free gun lock and safety** information: Project ChildSafe Safety Kit https://projectchildsafe.org/safety/get-a-safety-kit/ (project child safe).

Homelessness

Runaway or Homeless Youth

• Call: **(800)-RUNAWAY (1-800-786-2929)** or Text: **66008.**

HIV Prevention

• "PrEP reduces the risk of getting HIV from sex by about 99% when taken as prescribed" (CDC PrEP).

• Planned Parenthood PrEP call **(800) 230-7526.**

• Ready, Set, PrEP offers free HIV PrEP to those who qualify: https://readysetprep.hiv.gov/

COVID

• We will be living with COVID for the foreseeable future.

• Prevention and prompt treatment will be key to reducing complications.

• To find COVID-19 vaccine locations near you: Search vaccines.gov, **text** your ZIP code to **438829**, or call **1-800-232-0233.**

• Need help finding a place to get medication? Call **1-800-232-0233** (TTY **888-720-7489**).

Cancer

• Routine screening exams are important for early detection and treatment of cancer for the best chance at survival.

• Adults American Cancer Society Cancer Helpline **800.227.2345.**

• Children National Children's Cancer Society (NCCS) 314.241.1600 or toll-free **800.5FAMILY** (800.532.6459).

End of Life

• Advanced Directives can make your desires known if you are unable to speak for yourself.

• To contact your local Area Agency on Aging, call **800-677-1116.**

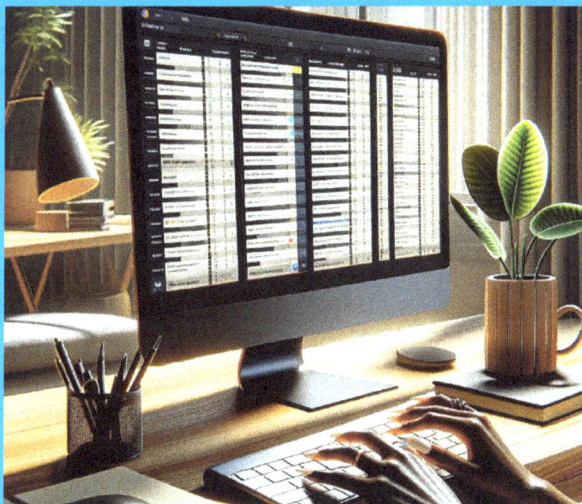

Author's Bio

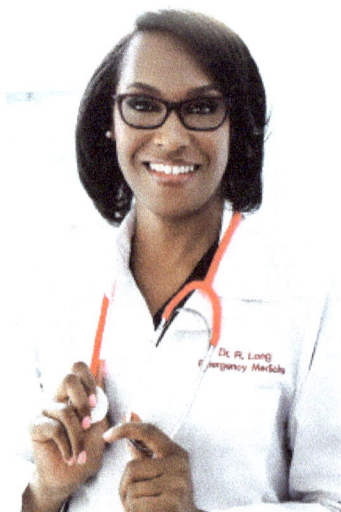

Dr. Ruby Long
THE CASUALTY DOC®

Dr. Long is a healer and advocate. She is a practitioner of Emergency Medicine and Restorative Justice Practices.

She is a graduate of Indiana University and Stanford Schools of Medicine for medical licensure and healthcare system leadership. She has completed the Restorative Justice Leadership Certificate of University of San Diego. Dr. Long is a Fellow of the American College of Emergency Physicians and has been board certified by the American Board of Emergency Medicine accreditation body.

In clinical practice, she addresses the acute life-threatening needs of individual patients before her in Emergency Departments (also known as the ER). In advocacy, she addresses the collective harm marginalized populations have experienced in accessing healthcare. This has included presenting implementation strategies in public hearing to the United States COVID-19 Health Equity Task Force.

Dr. Long is really a human being who has been in the positions of patient, worried family member and professional healthcare provider. Dr. Long is an avid traveler. She's a proud momma of a young son and all of his friends. She looks forward to the day that each human being can truly live their fullest life of happiness, health and authenticity.

She extends the greatest thanks to the village of biological and community parents who raised and loved on her, especially the FOLKS THAT DIDN'T SMASH HER DREAMS.

Stay in touch,
support@LoveLettersToPatients.org

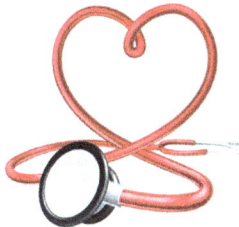

References

• AARI. Facts on Addiction and Opioids. AARI. 2020.
https://www.arlingtonva.us/Government/Programs/Health/Arling-
ton-Addiction-Recovery-Initiative/WhatareOpioids#:~:text=Some%20
opioids%20are%20used%20medically,by%20using%20opioid%20pain%20
relievers. Accessed December 2023.

• African Proverb, Reupert A. It Takes a Village to Raise a Child: Un-
derstanding and Expanding the Concept of the "Village." Front. Public
Health. March 2022.10. Doi.org/10.3389/fpubh.2022.756066. Accessed
October 20, 2023.

• Accessed December 2023. African Proverb, Reupert A. It Takes a
Village to Raise a Child: Understanding and Expanding the Concept of
the "Village." Front. Public Health. March 2022.10. Doi.org/10.3389/
fpubh.2022.756066. Accessed October 20, 2023.

• Ahmad F, Cisewski J, Xu J, Anderson R. Provisional Mortality Data
— United States, 2022. MMWR Morb Mortal Wkly Rep May 2023;
72:488–492. DOI: http://dx.doi.org/10.15585/mmwr.mm7218a3.

• Alio A, et al. Assessing the impact of paternal involvement on racial/
ethnic disparities in infant mortality rates. J Community Health. February 2011;36(1):63-8. doi: 10.1007/s10900-010-9280-3.

• American Academy of Dermatology (AAD). Skin Cancer In People
Of Color. AAD. 2024.
https://www.aad.org/public/diseases/skin-cancer/types/common/mel-
anoma/skin-color#:~: text=People%20of%20all%20colors%2C%20in-
cluding,cancer%20that%20can%20spread%20qui ckly. Accessed January
6, 2024.

• AAMC. Restorative Justice Academic Medicine (RJAM). AAMC. February 2023. Washington D.C.
https://cloud.email.aamc.org/RJAM. Accessed February 23, 2023.

• ACOG: Committee on Obstetric Practice. 731.
https://www.acog.org/clinical/clinical-guidance/committee-opinion/articles/2018/03/group-prenatal-care. Accessed August 31, 2022.

• Alberta. Learning About Hand-Foot Syndrome From Chemotherapy. MyHealthAlberta.CA Network. March 2023.
https://myhealth.alberta.ca/Health/aftercareinformation/pages/conditions.aspx?hwid=abq1892. Accessed September 24, 2023.

• Ali Center. In His Own Words. Muhammad Ali Museum and Education Center. 2024.
https://alicenter.org/meet-ali/in-his-own-words/. Accessed March 22, 2024.

• American Cancer Society (ACS). Can Childhood Cancers Be Prevented (Childhood CA)? 2022. American Cancer Society, Inc.
https://www.cancer.org/cancer/cancer-in-children/preventing-childhood-cancers.html. Accessed September 21, 2022.

• American Cancer Society (ACS). Caregiver Resource Guide. 2022. American Cancer Society, Inc.
https://www.cancer.org/treatment/caregivers/caregiver-resource-guide.html. Accessed September 24, 2022.

• American Cancer Society (ACS Cerv). Risk Factors for Cervical Cancer. ACS. January 2020.
https://www.cancer.org/cancer/types/cervical-cancer/causes-risks-prevention/risk-factors.html#:~:text=Women%20who%20smoke%20are%20about,the%20development%20of%20cervical %20cancer. Accessed March 22, 2024.

• American Cancer Society (ACS D). American Cancer Society Guidelines for the Early Detection of Cancer. 2022.
https://www.cancer.org/healthy/find-cancer-early/american-cancer-society-guidelines-for-the- early-detection-of-cancer.html. Accessed September 7, 2023.

• American Cancer Society (ACS Childhood). Can Childhood Cancers Be Prevented? ACS. October 2019.
https://www.cancer.org/cancer/types/cancer-in-children/preventing-childhood-cancers.html. Accessed September 21, 2022.

• American Cancer Society (ACS Key Stats). Key Statistics for Childhood Cancers. ACS. 2022.
https://www.cancer.org/cancer/cancer-in-children/key-statistics.html. Accessed September 21, 2022.

• American Cancer Society (ACS). Caregiver Resource Guide. ACS. 2024.
https://www.cancer.org/treatment/caregivers/caregiver-resource-guide.html. Access March 22, 2024.

• American Cancer Society (ACS S). Cancer Screening Recommendations. ACS. 2024.
https://www.cancer.org/cancer/screening/get-screened.html?gad=1&gclid=EAIaIQobChMI7p2o- MWZgQMVFCvUAR1pxgPlEAAYASAAEg-Jb0_D_BwE. Accessed March 22, 2024.

• American Cancer Society (ACS Staging). Cancer Staging. ACS. February 2022.
https://www.cancer.org/treatment/understanding-your-diagnosis/staging.html. Accessed October 1, 2022.

• American Cancer Society (ACS B). Changes in Memory, Thinking, and Focus (Chemo Brain). ACS. March 2024.
https://www.cancer.org/treatment/treatments-and-side-effects/physical-side-effects/changes-in- mood-or-thinking/chemo-brain.html. Accessed March 22, 2024.

• American Cancer Society (ACS E). Coping with Emotions as You Near the End of Life. May 2019.
https://www.cancer.org/treatment/end-of-life-care/nearing-the-end-of-life/emotions.html. Accessed September 30, 2022.

• American Cancer Society (ACS). Helping Children When a Family Member or Someone They Know Has Cancer. 2022.
https://www.cancer.org/treatment/children-and-cancer/when-a-family-member-has-cancer. html. Accessed September 30, 2022.

• American Cancer Society (ACS Non). Non-medical Treatments for Pain. January 2019.
https://www.cancer.org/treatment/treatments-and-side-effects/phys-ical-side-effects/pain/non-medical-treatments- for-cancer-pain.html. Accessed September 30, 2022.

• American Cancer Society (ACS Treating). Treating Children with Cancer. ACS. 2022.
https://www.cancer.org/cancer/cancer-in-children/how-are-childhood-cancers-treated.html. Accessed questions-about-indoor-air-and-coro-navirus-covid-19. Accessed September 29, 2022.

• AARI. Facts on Addiction and Opioids. AARI. 2020.
https://www.arlingtonva.us/Government/Programs/Health/Arling-ton-Addiction-Recovery-Initiative/Whatare-Opioids#:~:text=Some%20opioids%20are%20used%20medically,by%20using%20opioid%20pain%20relievers. Accessed December 2023.

• African Proverb, Reupert A. It Takes a Village to Raise a Child: Un-derstanding and Expanding the Concept of the "Village." Front. Public Health. March 2022.10. Doi.org/10.3389/fpubh.2022.756066. Accessed October 20, 2023.

• Ahmad F, Cisewski J, Xu J, Anderson R. Provisional Mortality Data — United States, 2022. MMWR Morb Mortal Wkly Rep May 2023; 72:488–492. DOI: http://dx.doi.org/10.15585/mmwr.mm7218a3.

• Alio A, et al. Assessing the impact of paternal involvement on racial/ethnic disparities in infant mortality rates. J Community Health. Febru-ary 2011;36(1):63-8. doi: 10.1007/s10900-010-9280-3.

• American Academy of Dermatology (AAD). Skin Cancer In People Of Color. AAD. 2024.
https://www.aad.org/public/diseases/skin-cancer/types/common/mela-noma/skincolor#:~:text=People%20of%20all%20colors%2C%20includ-ing,cancer%20that%20can%20spread%20qui
ckly. Accessed January 6, 2024.

• AAMC. Restorative Justice Academic Medicine (RJAM). AAMC. February 2023. Washington D.C. https://cloud.email.aamc.org/RJAM. Accessed February 23, 2023.

• ACOG: Committee on Obstetric Practice. 731. https://www.acog.org/clinical/clinical-guidance/committeeopinion/articles/2018/03/group-prenatal-care. Accessed August 31, 2022.

• Alberta. Learning About Hand-Foot Syndrome From Chemotherapy. MyHealthAlberta.CA Network. March 2023. https://myhealth.alberta.ca/Health/aftercareinformation/pages/conditions.aspx?hwid=abq1892. Accessed September 24, 2023.

• Ali Center. In His Own Words. Muhammad Ali Museum and Education Center. 2024. https://alicenter.org/meet-ali/in-his-own-words/. Accessed March 22, 2024.

• American Cancer Society (ACS). Can Childhood Cancers Be Prevented (Childhood CA)? 2022. American Cancer Society, Inc. https://www.cancer.org/cancer/cancer-in-children/preventing-childhood-cancers.html. Accessed September 21, 2022.

• American Cancer Society (ACS). Caregiver Resource Guide. 2022. American Cancer Society, Inc. https://www.cancer.org/treatment/caregivers/caregiver-resource-guide.html. Accessed September 24, 2022.

• American Cancer Society (ACS Cerv). Risk Factors for Cervical Cancer. ACS. January 2020. https://www.cancer.org/cancer/types/cervical-cancer/causes-risks-prevention/riskfactors.html#:~:text=Women%20who%20smoke%20are%20about,the%20development%20of%20cervical%20cancer. Accessed March 22, 2024.

• American Cancer Society (ACS D). American Cancer Society Guidelines for the Early Detection of Cancer. 2022. https://www.cancer.org/healthy/find-cancer-early/american-cancer-society-guidelines-forthe-early-detection-of-cancer.html. Accessed September 7, 2023.

• American Cancer Society (ACS Childhood). Can Childhood Cancers Be Prevented? ACS. October 2019. https://www.cancer.org/cancer/types/cancer-in-children/preventing-childhood-cancers.html. Accessed September 21, 2022.

• American Cancer Society (ACS Key Stats). Key Statistics for Childhood Cancers. ACS. 2022. https://www.cancer.org/cancer/cancer-in-children/key-statistics.html Accessed September 21, 2022.

• American Cancer Society (ACS). Caregiver Resource Guide. ACS. 2024. https://www.cancer.org/treatment/caregivers/caregiver-resource-guide.html. Accessed March 22, 2024.

• American Cancer Society (ACS S). Cancer Screening Recommendations. ACS. 2024. https://www.cancer.org/cancer/screening/get-screened.html?gad=1&gclid=EAIaIQobChMI7p2o-MWZgQMVFCvUAR1pxgPIEAAYA-SAAEgJb0_D_BwE. Accessed March 22, 2024.

• American Cancer Society (ACS Staging). Cancer Staging. ACS. February 2022. https://www.cancer.org/treatment/understanding-your-diagnosis/staging.html. Accessed October 1, 2022.

• American Cancer Society (ACS B). Changes in Memory, Thinking, and Focus (Chemo Brain). ACS. March 2024. https://www.cancer.org/treatment/treatments-and-side-effects/physical-side-effects/changesin-mood-or-thinking/chemo-brain.html. Accessed March 22, 2024.

• American Cancer Society (ACS E). Coping with Emotions as You Near the End of Life. May 2019. https://www.cancer.org/treatment/end-of-life-care/nearing-the-end-of-life/emotions.html. Accessed September 30, 2022.

• American Cancer Society (ACS). Helping Children When a Family Member or Someone They Know Has Cancer. 2022. https://www.cancer.org/treatment/children-and-cancer/when-a-family-member-hascancer.html. Accessed September 30, 2022.

• American Cancer Society (ACS Non). Non-medical Treatments for Pain. January 2019.
https://www.cancer.org/treatment/treatments-and-side-effects/phys-ical-side-effects/pain/non-medicaltreatments-for-cancer-pain.html. Accessed September 30, 2022.

• American Cancer Society (ACS Treating). Treating Children with Cancer. ACS. 2022.
https://www.cancer.org/cancer/cancer-in-children/how-are-childhood-cancers-treated.html. Accessed September 21, 2022.

• American Cancer Society (ACS H). What is Hospice Care? ACS. May 2019.
https://www.cancer.org/treatment/end-of-life-care/hospice-care/what-is-hospice-care.html. Accessed September 30, 2022.

• American Cancer Society (ACS). When Your Child Has Cancer. 2022. American Cancer Society, Inc.
https://www.cancer.org/treatment/children-and-cancer/when-your-child-has-cancer.html. Accessed September 21, 2022.

• American Cancer Society (ACS Pro). American Cancer Society Recommendations for Prostate Cancer Early Detection. ACS. November 2023.
https://www.cancer.org/cancer/prostate-cancer/detectiondiagnosis-staging/acsrecommendations.html#:~:text=The%20discussion%20about%20screening%20should,risk%20of%20developing%20pros-tate%20cancer. Accessed March 22, 2024.

• American Cancer Society (ACS P) Where Is Hospice Care Provided and How Is It Paid For?. ACS. December 2023.
https://www.cancer.org/cancer/end-of-life-care/hospice-care/who-pro-vides-hospicecare.html. Accessed March 22, 2024.

• ACOG Committee on Obstetric Practice (ACOG GPC). ACOG Committee Opinion Number 731: Group Prenatal Care. Obstetrics & Gynecology. March 2018. 131 (3). E104-108.

• ACOG District II (ACOG II). Maternal Safety Bundle for Obstetric Hemorrhage. Safe Motherhood Initiative. ACOG. January 2020.
https://www.acog.org/-/media/project/acog/acogorg/files/forms/districts/smi-ob-hemorrhage-bundle-slides.pdf. Accessed October 20, 2023.

• American College of Obstetricians and Gynecologist (ACOG Mamm). ACOG Revises Breast Cancer Screening Guidance: Ob-Gyns Promote Shared Decision Making. ACOG. June 2017. https://www.acog.org/news/news-releases/2017/06/acog-revises-breast-cancer-screening-guidance-obgyns-promote-shared-decision-making. Accessed March 22, 2024.

• American College of Obstetricians and Gynecologist (ACOG Elim). Eliminating Preventable Maternal Mortality and Morbidity. ACOG. 2023. https://www.acog.org/advocacy/policy-priorities/maternalmortality-prevention. Accessed October 20, 2023.

• American College of Obstetricians and Gynecologist (ACOG Gun V). Gun Violence and Safety. ACOG. February 2019. https://www.acog.org/clinical-information/polcy-and-position-statements/statements-ofpolicy/2019/gun-violence-and-safety. Accessed October 20, 2023.

• American College of Obstetricians and Gynecologist (ACOG Cerv). Updated Cervical Cancer Screening Guidelines. ACOG. April 2021. https://www.acog.org/clinical/clinical-guidance/practiceadvisory/articles/2021/04/updated-cervical-cancer-screening-guidelines. Accessed March 22, 2024.

• ADANN. Health Care and the Americans With Disabilities Act. ADANN. March 2024. https://adata.org/factsheet/health-care-and-ada. Accessed March 22, 2024.

• ADANN (ADANN Aux). What kinds of auxiliary aids and services are required by the ADA to ensure effective communication with individuals with hearing or vision impairments?. ADANN. March 2024. https://adata.org/faq/what-kinds-auxiliary-aids-and-services-are-required-ada-ensure-effectivecommunication. Accessed March 22, 2024.

• Adler D. Reed v. Reed and the Fight for Gender Equality. Territory. November 2017.
https://territorymag.com/articles/reed-v-reed-fight-genderequality/#:~:-text=for%20women's%20rights.-,Reed%20v.,his%20father's%20base-ment%20in%20Boise. Accessed October 10, 2023.

• Akbulut N, Razum O. Why Othering should be considered in research on health inequalities: Theoretical perspectives and research needs. SSM Popul Health. 2022 Nov 5;20:101286. doi:10.1016/j.ss-mph.2022.101286. PMID: 36406107.

• Akkas F. Suicides During and Shortly After Pregnancy Are an Urgent Concern. Pew Charitable Trusts. October 2022.
https://www.pewtrusts.org/en/research-and-analysis/arcles/2022/10/06/suicides-duringand-shortly-after-pregnancy-are-an-urgent-concern. Accessed October 20, 2023.

• Amanik A, Fletcher K. Till Death Do Us Part: American Ethnic Cemeteries as Borders Uncrossed. University Press of Mississippi. 2020. Doi.org/10.14325/mississippi/9781496827883.001.0001.

• American Heart Association (AHA Stroke). About Stroke. 2022. https://www.stroke.org/en/about-stroke. Accessed September 22, 2024.

• American Heart Association (HFCause). Causes and Risks for Heart Failure. May 2017.
https://www.heart.org/en/health-topics/heart-failure/causes-and-risks-for-heart-failure. Accessed October 1, 2022.

• American Heart Association (HFDevices). Devices and Surgical Procedures to Treat Heart Failure. July 2023.
https://www.heart.org/en/health-topics/heart-failure/treatment-options-for-heart-failure/devices-andsurgical-procedures-to-treat-heart-failure. Accessed September 22, 2023.

• American Heart Association. (AHA Maternity) Heart health is sub-optimal among American Indian/Alaska Native women, supports needed. AHA. May 2023.
https://newsroom.heart.org/news/heart-health-is-suboptimal-among-

american-indianalaska-native-women-supports-needed. Accessed October 20, 2023.

• American Heart Association (HFMeds). Medications Used to Treat Heart Failure. AHA. July 2023.
https://www.heart.org/en/health-topics/heart-failure/treatment-options-for-heart-failure/medications-usedto-treat-heart-failure. Accessed October 1, 2023.

• American Heart Association News (AHA S). Stroke symptoms require emergency treatment even if they quickly disappear, new report says. AHA. January 2023.
https://www.heart.org/en/news/2023/01/19/strokesymptoms-require-emergency-treatment-even-if-they-quickly-disappear-new-report-says. Accessed March 24, 2024.

• December 2022.
https://www.heart.org/en/health-topics/heart-attack/about-heart-attacks. Accessed September 22, 2023.

• American Heart Association (HF). What is Heart Failure. March 2023. https://www.heart.org/en/healthtopics/heart-failure/what-is-heart-failure. Accessed September 22, 2023.

• American Heart Association (AHA TIA). What is a TIA. 2018. https://www.stroke.org/en/aboutstroke/types-of-stroke/tia-transient-ischemic-attack/what-is-a-tia. Accessed September 22, 2023.

• American Heart Association (AHA T). Why Getting Quick Stroke Treatment is Important. June 2021.
https://www.stroke.org/en/about-stroke/types-of-stroke/is-getting-quick-stroke-treatment-important. Accessed October 20, 2023.

• American Heart Association (AHA Newsroom). Women found to be at higher risk for heart failure and heart attack death than men. November 2020.
https://newsroom.heart.org/news/women-found-to-be-athigher-risk-for-heart-failure-and-heart-attack-death-than-men Accessed September 22, 2023.

• American Lung Association (ALA). Lung Cancer Causes & Risk Factors. ALA. November 2022.
https://www.lung.org/lung-health-diseases/lung-disease-lookup/lung-cancer/basics/what-causes-lungcancer. Accessed January 10, 2024.

• American Stroke Association (AStroke). ACT F.A.S.T. Tip Sheet. AStroke. 2023.
https://www.stroke.org/en/about-stroke/stroke-symptoms. Accessed October 20, 2023.

• Andersson E, Small R. Fathers' satisfaction with two different models of antenatal care in Sweden-Findings from a quasi-experimental study. Midwifery. July 2017;50:201-207. doi:10.1016/j.midw.2017.04.014. Epub 2017 Apr 29. PMID: 28475916.

• Andino I. Why It Works. radical Health. July 2017. https://www.radical-health.com/why-it-works. Accessed September 10, 2022.

• Artiga S., Hinton E. Beyond Health Care: The Role of Social Determinants in Promoting Health and Health Equity. KFF. May 2018.
https://www.kff.org/racial-equity-and-health-policy/issue-brief/beyond-healthcare-the-role-of-social-determinants-in-promoting-health-and-health-equity/. Accessed October 20, 2023.

• ASPR. Find Covid Meds. ASPR. 2022.
https://covid-19-test-to-treat-locator-dhhs.hub.arcgis.com/. Accessed October 20, 2023.

• Aubrey A. If you're 40, it's time to start mammograms, according to new guidelines. NPR. May 2023.
https://www.npr.org/sections/health-shots/2023/05/09/1174167602/if-youre-40-its-time-to-startmammograms-according-to-new-guidelines. Accessed March 22, 2024.

• Barnett W, Burke Harris N. Investing Early. The Burke Foundation. 2018.
https://burkefoundation.org/what-drives-us/investing-early/. Accessed October 20, 2023.

• Barry D, Brown S. Nipsey Hussle, Gun Violence and the Big Business of Weapons. April 2019.
https://sdvoice.info/nipsey-hussle-gun-violence-and-the-big-business-of-weapons/. Accessed October 20, 2023.

• Behel J. I shall be released. Restorative justice techniques can address healthcare burnout & attrition. Reflective MedEd. 2019.

• Bhushan D, Kotz K, McCall J, Wirtz S, Gilgoff R, Dube SR, Powers C, Olson-Morgan J, Galeste M, Patterson K, Harris L, Mills A, Bethell C, Burke Harris N, Office of the California Surgeon General. Roadmap for Resilience: The California Surgeon General's Report on Adverse Childhood Experiences, Toxic Stress, and Health. Office of the California Surgeon General, 2020. DOI: 10.48019/PEAM8812.

• BMJ. Homicide is a leading cause of death in pregnant women in the US. The BMJ. 2023.
https://www.bmj.com/company/newsroom/homicide-is-a-leading-cause-of-death-in-pregnant-women-intheus/#:~:text=Homicide%20is%20a%20leading%20cause%20of%20death%20in%20pregnant%20women%20in%20the%20US,-BMJ&text=Women%20in%20the%20US%20are,experts%20in%20The%20BMJ%20today. Accessed October 20, 2023.

• Boyes-Watson C, Pranis K. Circle Forward Revised Edition 2020. Living Justice Press. 2020. ISBN 978-1-937141-19-6.

• Boyle P. Threats against health care workers are rising. Here's how hospitals are protecting their staffs. AAMC News. August 2022.
https://www.aamc.org/news/threats-against-health-care-workers-are-risingheres-how-hospitals-are-protecting-their-staffs. Accessed March 22, 2024.

• Boyle P. What is gender-affirming care? Your questions answered. AAMC News. April 2022.
https://www.aamc.org/news/what-gender-affirming-care-your-questions-answered. Accessed August 25, 2022.

• Bridger H, Skin Tone and Pulse Oximetry Racial disparities in care tied to differences in pulse oximeter performance. Harvard Medical School. July 2022.
https://hms.harvard.edu/news/skin-tone-pulse-oximetry

• Braun H, et. al. Cancer in Transgender People: Evidence and Methodological Considerations. Epidemiol Rev. January 2017; 39(1):93-107. doi: 10.1093/epirev/mxw003.

• Brueck H, Cheng J. These are the US states where people live the longest, healthiest lives — and the shortest. Business Insider. April 2018. https://www.businessinsider.com/ranked-life-expectancy-by-state-2018-4. Accessed October 20, 2023.

• Bullard R. Articles: Enviornmental Justice. Dr. Robert Bullard: Father of Environmental Justice.
https://drrobertbullard.com/articles/. Accessed October 20, 2023.

• Burke Harris N. About: The Burke Foundation. Burke Foundation. 2022. https://burkefoundation.org/whatdrives-us/adverse-childhood-experiences-aces/. Accessed September13, 2022.

• Burke Harris N, Raz G. Nadine Burke Harris: How Does Trauma Affect A Child's DNA? NPR. August 2017.
https://www.npr.org/transcripts/545092982. Accessed October 20, 2023.

• Burns A. Long COVID: What Do the Latest Data Show? KFF. January 2023.
https://www.kff.org/policywatch/long-covid-what-do-latest-data-show/. Accessed November 2, 2023.

• Byerley, B.M., Haas, D.M. A systematic overview of the literature regarding group prenatal care for highrisk pregnant women. BMC Pregnancy Childbirth 17, 329 (2017).
https://doi.org/10.1186/s12884-017-1522-2

• Canales M. Othering: toward an understanding of difference. ANS Adv Nurs Sci. June 2000;22(4):16-31.doi: 10.1097/00012272-200006000-00003. PMID: 10852666.

• Cancer Care. Caregiving at the end of life. Cancer Care. February 2022. https://www.cancercare.org/publications/63-caregiving_at_the_end_ of_life Accessed September 30, 2022.

• Centers for Disease Control and Prevention (CDC ACEs). Adverse Childhood Experiences (ACEs). CDC. June 2023. https://www.cdc.gov/violenceprevention/aces/index.html. Accessed October 20, 2023.

• Centers for Disease Control and Prevention (CDC:ANV). A New View of Life Expectancy .CDC. March 2020. https://www.cdc.gov/surveillance/blogs-stories/life-expectancy.html. Accessed October 20, 2023.

• Centers for Disease Control and Prevention (CDC B). Basics of COVID-19. November 2021. https://www.cdc.gov/coronavirus/2019-ncov/your-health/about-covid-19/basics-covid-19.html. Accessed October 2, 2022.

• Centers for Disease Control and Prevention (CDC Data). COVID-19 Monthly Death Rates per 100,000 Population by Age Group, Race and Ethnicity, and Sex. CDC. November 2023. https://covid.cdc.gov/covid-data-tracker/#demographicsovertime. Accessed December 13, 2023.

• Centers for Disease Control and Prevention (CDC COVID Treatment Med). COVID-19 Treatments and Medications. CDC. March 2024. https://www.cdc.gov/coronavirus/2019-ncov/your-health/treat-ments-forsevere-illness.html.Accessed March 22, 2024.

• Centers for Disease Control and Prevention (CDC D). Disability Impacts All of Us. CDC. May 2023. Accessed March 22, 2024.

• Centers for Disease Control and Prevention (CDC Heart). Heart Disease Facts. May 2023. https://www.cdc.gov/heartdisease/facts.htm Accessed September 22, 2023.

• Centers for Disease Control and Prevention (CDC). Heart Failure. 2020. https://www.cdc.gov/heartdisease/heart_failure.htm. Accessed September 22, 2022.

• Centers for Disease Control and Prevention CDC (CDC Prep). HIV: PrEP Effectiveness. CDC. June 2022. https://www.cdc.gov/hiv/basics/prep/prep-effectiveness.html. Accessed July 27, 2022.

• Centers for Disease Control and Prevention (CDC Kinds). Kinds of Cancer. CDC. August 2023. https://www.cdc.gov/cancer/kinds.htm#:~:text=Skin%20cancer%20is%20the%20most%20common%20cancer%20in%20the%20United%20States. Accessed March 22, 2024.

• Centers for Disease Control and Prevention (CDC LD). Leading Causes of Death. National Center for Health Statistics. January 2024. https://www.cdc.gov/nchs/fastats/leading-causes-of-death.htm. Accessed March 22, 2024.

• Centers for Disease Control and Prevention (CDC L). Life Expectancy. National Center for Health Statistics. February 2023. https://www.cdc.gov/nchs/fastats/life-expectancy.htm. Accessed March 22, 2024.

• Centers for Disease Control and Prevention (CDC LE). Life Expectancy in the U.S. Dropped for the Second Year in a Row in 2021. CDC. August 2022. https://www.cdc.gov/nchs/pressroom/nchs_press_releases/2022/20220831.html. Accessed October 1, 2022.

• Centers for Disease Control and Prevention (CDC LC). Long COVID or Post-COVID Conditions. CDC. March 2024. https://www.cdc.gov/coronavirus/2019-ncov/long-term-effects/index.html. Accessed March 21, 2024.

• Centers for Disease Control and Prevention (PMSS). Pregnancy Mortality Surveillance System (PMSS). CDC. June 2022. https://www.cdc.gov/reproductivehealth/maternal-mortality/pregnancy-mortalitysurveillance-system.htm. Accessed September 1, 2022.

• Centers for Disease Control and Prevention. STI. Jan 2021.
https://www.cdc.gov/media/releases/2021/p0125-sexualy-transmit-
ted-infection.html. Accessed October 14, 2022.

• Centers for Disease Control and Prevention (CDC SB). Science
Brief: SARS-CO-V-2. CDC. April 2021.
https://www.cdc.gov/coronavirus/2019-ncov/more/science-and-re-
search/surfacetransmission.html#:~:text=Data%20from%20surface%20
survival%20studies,%2C%2012%2C%2013%2C%2015.
Accessed September 29, 2022.

• Centers for Disease Control and Prevention (CDC Stroke). About
Stroke. CDC. May 2023.
https://www.cdc.gov/stroke/about.htm. Accessed October 20, 2023.

• Centers for Disease Control and Prevention (CDC Sun). Sun Safety.
April 2022.
https://www.cdc.gov/cancer/skin/basic_info/sun-safety.htm. Accessed
September 26, 2022.

• Centers for Disease Control and Prevention (CDC C19). Symptoms
of COVID-19. CDC. March 2024.
https://www.cdc.gov/coronavirus/2019-ncov/symptoms-testing/symp-
toms.html. Accessed March 22, 2024.

• Centers for Disease Control and Prevention (CDC Covid Treatment Med). COVID-19 Treatments and Medications. CDC. March 2024.
https://www.cdc.gov/coronavirus/2019-ncov/your-health/treat-
ments-forsevere-illness.html. Accessed March 22, 2024.

• Centers for Disease Control and Prevention (CDC Violence
Prevention). Violence Prevention: Fast Facts: Violence Prevention. CDC.
May 2022.
https://www.cdc.gov/violenceprevention/firearms/fastfact.html.
Accessed September 21, 2022.

• Centers for Disease Control and Prevention. What are the Risk
Factors for Skin Cancer. April 2022.
https://www.cdc.gov/cancer/skin/basic_info/risk_factors.html. Accessed
September 26, 2022.

• Center for Ethical Leadership (CEL). About Peacemaking & Healing Circles. Center for Ethical Leadership. 2016. https://www.ethicalleadership.org/peacemaking-circles.html. Accessed August 11, 2023.

• Centers for Disease Control and Prevention Blog Administrator (CDC TIC). Building Trauma-Informed Communities. CDC. May 2022. https://blogs.cdc.gov/publichealthmatters/2022/05/trauma-informed/. Accessed October 20, 2023.

• Center for Restorative Justice (CRJ). Rx for RJ. University of San Diego. December 2017. https://www.sandiego.edu/soles/centers-and-institutes/restorative-justice/initiatives/#:~:text=Tailored%20specifically%20for%20the%20unique,learner%20mistreatment%20and%20provide%20a. Accessed September 2020.

• Cheng E. et al. The Influence of Antenatal Partner Support on Pregnancy Outcomes. J Womens Health (Larchmt). July 2016;25(7):672-9. doi: 10.1089/jwh.2015.5462.

• Child Mind, Jacobson R. Helping Kids Who Are Scared of Going to the Doctor. Child Mind Institute.October 2023. Accessed March 22, 2024.

• Christensen J. For gunshot survivors, recovery can last a lifetime. CNN. June 2016. https://www.cnn.com/2016/06/17/health/gunshot-wound-long-recovery/index.html. Accessed September 26, 2022.

• Clare M. Mother who survived attack wants public to know about progression of domestic violence. KSAT12. June 2023. https://www.youtube.com/watch?v=YnxAJrH8wsM. Accessed October 20, 2023.

• Coleman A. 'Hundreds dead' because of Covid-19 misinformation. BBC. August 2020. https://www.bbc.com/news/world-53755067. Access December 11, 2023.

• Cohen J, West B. RBG. Magnolia Pictures and Participant Media. 2018. Film.

• Coussons-Read M. Effects of prenatal stress on pregnancy and human development: mechanisms and pathways. Obstet Med. 2013 Jun;6(2):52-57. doi: 10.1177/1753495X12473751.

• Cross D, Burmester JK. Gene therapy for cancer treatment: past, present and future. Clin Med Res. September 2006. 4(3):218-27. doi: 10.3121/cmr.4.3.218.

• Cunningham SD, Lewis JB, Shebl FM, Boyd LM, Robinson MA, Grilo SA, Lewis SM, Pruett AL, Ickovics JR. Group Prenatal Care Reduces Risk of Preterm Birth and Low Birth Weight: A Matched Cohort Study. J Womens Health (Larchmt). 2019 Jan;28(1):17-22. doi: 10.1089/jwh.2017.6817. Epub 2018 Sep 25. PMID:30256700.

• Darling J. EDU-X785R Introduction to Restorative Justice: A Global Social Movement. University of San Diego. July 2021.

• Davis F, Jenkins M. "What is Justice?" With Fania Davis and Morris Jenkins. World Trust. June 2016.
https://www.youtube.com/watch?v=PE6B1N_-rC8. Accessed October 20, 2023.

• Davis F. Little Book of Race and Restorative Justice: Black Lives, Healing, and US Social Transformation. Good Books. April 2019. ISBN-13: 978-1680993431.

• Dawson K. Diabetes care in First Nations populations in British Columbia. BC Medical Journal. Novembe 2018; (60) 9: 451-454.

• Deutsch M. Creating a safe and welcoming clinic environment. UCSF. June 2016.
https://transcare.ucsf.edu/guidelines/clinic-environment. Accessed August 26, 2022.

• Drake P, Rudowiz R. Tracking Social Determinants of Health During the COVID-19 Pandemic. April 2022.
https://www.kff.org/coronavirus-covid-19/issue-brief/tracking-social-determinants-of-health-duringthe-covid-19-pandemic/. Accessed October 20, 2023.

• Eligon J. Black Doctor Dies of Covid-19 After Complaining of Racist Treatment. New York Times. December 2020.
https://www.nytimes.com/2020/12/23/us/susan-moore-black-doctor-indiana.html. Accessed October 20, 2023.

• Equal Justice Initiative (EJI). Healthcare. EJI. 2023. https://eji.org/projects/health-care/. Accessed October 20, 2023.

• Enomoto C. 'n Dis Life' Israel touched many. June 1997. Honolulu Star Bulletin.
https://archives.starbulletin.com/1997/06/27/features/story1.html. Accessed January 16, 2024.

• EPA. Frequently Questions about Indoor Air and Coronavirus (COVID-19). EPA. December 2021.
https://www.epa.gov/coronavirus/frequent-questions-about-indoor-air-and-coronavirus-covid-19. Accessed September 29, 2022.

• EPA. Indoor Air and Coronavirus (COVID-19) EPA December 2021.
https://www.epa.gov/coronavirus/indoor-air-and-coronavirus-covid-19#:~:text=Transmission%20of%20COVID%2D19%20from,for%20hours%20in%20some%20cases. Accessed September 29, 2022.

• Everytown. Guns and Violence Against Women. Everytown Research & Policy. April 2023.
https://everytownresearch.org/report/guns-and-violence-against-women-americas-uniquely-lethal-intimatepartner-violenceproblem/#:~:text=Intimate%20partner%20gun%20violence%20makes,were%20from%20the%20United%20States. Accessed October 20, 2023.

• Family Search (FS). Evangeline L. Kamakawiwo'ole. FS. 2021.
https://ancestors.familysearch.org/en/L2MP-X34/evangeline-l.-kamakawiwo%27ole-1966-1987. Accessed October 10, 2023.

• Federal Drug Administration (EUA). Emergency Use Authorization. FDA. March 2024.
https://www.fda.gov/emergency-preparedness-and-response/mcm-legal-regulatory-and-policyframework/emergency-use-authorization. Accessed March 22, 2024.

• Federal Drug Administration (FDA). Know Your Treatment Options. FDA. December 2023.
https://www.fda.gov/consumers/consumer-updates/know-your-treatment-options-covid-19. Accessed March 22, 2024.

• Feke T. What's the Difference Between Palliative Care and Hospice? Very Well. February 2024.
https://www.verywellhealth.com/palliative-care-vs-hospice-7090656. Accessed March 22, 2024.

• Felitti V, et al. Relationship of childhood abuse and household dysfunction to many of the leading causes of death in adults. The Adverse Childhood Experiences (ACE) Study. Am J Prev Med. 1998 May;14(4):245-58. doi: 10.1016/s0749-3797(98)00017-8. PMID: 9635069.

• Felitti V. The Relation Between Adverse Childhood Experiences and Adult Health: Turning Gold into
Lead. Perm J. 2002 Winter;6(1):44-47. doi: 10.7812/TPP/02.994. PMID: 30313011.

• Fenway Health. New Study Finds Significant Barriers To Gender-Affirming Primary Care Among Transgender People Living In Rural Areas. Fenway Health. August 2022. https://fenwayhealth.org/newstudy-finds-significant-barriers-to-gender-affirming-primry-care-among-transgender-people-living-inrural-areas/. Accessed October 17, 2022.

• Find A Grave (Grave). Evangeline Leinani "Angie" Keale Kamakawiwo'ole. Grave. March 2000.
https://www.findagrave.com/memorial/3780121/evangeline-leinani-kamakawiwo'ole. Accessed October 10, 2023.

• Find A Grave (Gravell). Henry Kaleialoha Naniwa "Tiny" Kamakawiwo'ole Jr. Grave. March 2000. https://www.findagrave.com/memorial/3780122/henry-kaleialoha_naniwa-kamakawiwo'ole. Accessed October 10, 2023.

• Fernald C, Kapusta J. Remebering RBG: A Look Back at the life and legacy of a legend, a year after her passing. Florida Bar Journal. January/February 2022; 96 (1) 30.

• Fletcher K. Fresh to Death: African Americans and RIP T-Shirts. Nursing Clio. August 2020. https://nursingclio.org/2020/08/13/fresh-to-death-african-americans-and-rip-t-shirts/. Accessed March 22, 2024.

• Ford E. Peace is a lifestyle. Life Camp. 2023. https://www.peaceisalifestyle.com/. Accessed October 20, 2023.

• Fortier J. An overdose drug is finally over-the-counter. Is that enough to stop the death toll? NPR. September 2023. https://www.npr.org/sections/health-shots/2023/09/26/1199371609/an-overdose-drug-isfinally-over-the-counter-is-that-enough-to-stop-the-death-to. Accessed October 20, 2023.

• Fragoso S. How Do We Heal? (With Resmaa Menakem). Talk Easy with Sam Fragoso Episode 200. November 2020. https://talkeasypod.com/resmaamenakem/#:~:text=%E2%80%9CMany%20times%20trauma%20in%20a,begin%20to%20discern%20what's%20what.%E2%80%9D. Accessed March 22, 2024.

• Frankl V. Man's Search for Meaning: An Introduction to Logotherapy. Boston. Beacon Press. 1962.

• Funes Y. The Father of Environmental Justice Exposes the Geography of Inequity. Nature. September 2023. https://www.nature.com/articles/d41586-023-02613-6. Accessed October 20, 2023.

• Gallagher W. Fentanyl-Laced Marijuana on the Rise. Claudia Black Young Adult Center. August 2023.
https://www.claudiablackcenter.com/fentanyl-laced-marijua-na-on-the-rise/. Accessed December 21, 2023.

• Gage Witvliet M. I've had COVID-19 for a year. Here's what I've learned. TEDx Mile High. March 2021.
https://www.youtube.com/watch?v=4LX_JRHZdkI. Accessed October 20, 2023.

• Garrett U. Luther Vandross, Celebrating the Legacy of a Legend. BET. August 2023.
https://www.bet.com/article/mta6ga/luther-vandross-celebrating-the-legend-music-spotlight. Accessed March 22, 2024.

• Geronimus A, et al. "Weathering" and age patterns of allostatic load scores among Blacks and Whites in the United States. Am J Public Health. May 2006; 96(5):826-33. doi: 10.2105/AJPH.2004.060749.

• Goldman-Mellor S, Margerison C. Maternal drug-related death and suicide are leading causes of postpartum death in California. Am J Obstet Gynecol. 2019 Nov;221(5):489.e1-489.e9. doi:10.1016/j.ajog.2019.05.045.

• Global Reference Group for Children (Global Ref). Affected by COVID-19. COVID-19–Associated Orphanhood and Caregiver Death in the United States. Imperial College London. June 2023.
https://imperialcollegelondon.github.io/orphanhood_USA/. Accessed March 22, 2024.

• Goldstick J, Cunningham R, Carter P. Current Causes of Death in Children and Adolescents in the United States. N Engl J Med. May 2022; 386:1955-1956. DOI: 10.1056/NEJMc2201761.

• GoodRx, Williams G. How to Get Free Narcan to Keep at Home. GoodRx Health. January 2022.
https://www.goodrx.com/naloxone/narcan-naloxone-at-home-free . Accessed August 22, 2022.

• Gottlieb E, Ziegler J, Morley K, Rush B, Celi LA. Assessment of Racial and Ethnic Differences in Oxygen Supplementation Among Patients in the Intensive Care Unit. JAMA Intern Med. July 2022;182(8):849–858. doi:10.1001/jamainternmed.2022.2587.

• Guidi J. et al. Allostatic Load and Its Impact on Health: A Systematic Review. Psychother Psychosom. December 2020; 90 (1): 11–27. Doi.org/10.1159/000510696.

• GW Cancer Center. I Want You to Know: Patient Cards in English, Spanish and Chinese. GWHS. https://cancercontroltap.smhs.gwu.edu/news/i-want-you-know. Accessed October 20, 2023.

• Hafeez H, et al. Health Care Disparities Among Lesbian, Gay, Bisexual, and Transgender Youth: A Literature Review. Cureus. Apr 2017;9(4):e1184. doi: 10.7759/cureus.1184. PMID: 28638747; PMCID.

• Hargarten S. Commentary: Moving Emergency Medicine Toward the Biopsychosocial Disease Model Annals of Emergency Medicine November 2019;74(5):S52-S54.

• Harvard Chan. Homicide leading cause of death for pregnant women in U.S. Harvard. 2022. https://www.hsph.harvard.edu/news/hsph-in-the-news/homicide-leading-cause-of-death-for-pregnantwomen-in-u-s/. Accessed March 22, 2024.

• Harvard Medical School (HMS). Skin Tone and Pulse Oximetry. HMS. July 2022. https://hms.harvard.edu/news/skin-tone-pulse-oximetry. Accessed March 22, 2024.

• Hassanein N. Preventable injuries are killing America's children. But some are more at risk than others. USA Today. February 2023. https://www.usatoday.com/story/news/health/2023/02/21/child-injuriesleading-cause-death-risk/11002455002/. Accessed October 20, 2023.

• HealthcareCAN, Richardson LMT. Bringing reconciliation to healthcare in Canada: wise practices forhealthcare leaders. HealthcareCAN. 2018.

• Healthpeople.gov. 2020 Topics & Objectives: Lesbian, Gay, Bisexual, and Transgender Health. ODPHP. February 2022.
https://www.healthypeople.gov/2020/topics-objectives/topic/lesbian-gay-bisexual-andtransgender-health. Accessed August 26, 2022.

• Henry Ford Health Staff. What Does COVID-19 Do To Your Body? Henry Ford. April 2020.
https://www.henryford.com/blog/2020/04/what-does-covid19-do-to-your-body. Accessed October 2, 2022.

• HHS. How do I report elder abuse or abuse of an older person or senior? HHS. March 2014.
https://www.hhs.gov/answers/programs-for-families-and-children/how-do-i-report-elder-abuse/index.html. Accessed October 20, 2023.

• Horovitz B. Death Doesn't Have To Be So Scary. KFF Health News. February 2017.
https://kffhealthnews.org/news/death-doesnt-have-to-be-so-scary/. Accessed October 20, 2023.

• Hospice Foundation of America (HFA). What is Hospice. HFA. 2022.
https://hospicefoundation.org/Hospice-Care/Hospice-Services. Accessed September 30, 2022.

• Howard Brown Health. Transgender and Gender Nonconforming Essentials. AMA Ed Hub. October 2020.
https://edhub.ama-assn.org/howard-brown-cme/interactive/18543812. Accessed August 25, 2022.

• Hoyert D. Maternal mortality rates in the United States, 2020. NCHS Health E-Stats. 2022. DOI:
https://dx.doi.org/10.15620/cdc:113967external icon. Accessed September 1, 2022.

• Hussle, Nipsey. The Hussle Way. Bullets Ain't Got No Name Vol. 3. All Money In Records, August 4, 2009.

• Indigenous Watchdog (IW). HealthcareCAN. Indigenous Watchdog. April 2018.
https://www.indigenouswatchdog.org/update/12427/. Accessed October 20, 2023.

• Izhawaii.com (IzBio). Iz® Biography (IzBio). The Official Site of Israel Kamakawiwoʻole.
https://izhawaii.com/biography/. Accessed February 13, 2024.

• Jackson S, et. al. Cancer Stage, Treatment, and Survival Among Transgender Patients in the United States. J Natl Cancer Inst. Septemeber 2021;113(9):1221-1227. doi: 10.1093/jnci/djab028.

• Jenkins, M. Gullah Island Dispute Resolution: An Example of Afrocentric Restorative Justice. Journal of Black Studies. Novemeber 2006. 37(2), 299-319. Doi.org/10.1177/0021934705277497.

• Jiang L, et. al. A Systematic Review of Persistent Clinical Features After SARS-CoV-2 in the Pediatric Population. Pediatrics. August 2023; 152 (2): e2022060351. 10.1542/peds.2022-060351.

• Johnson S, Sabo S. New Census Bureau Population Estimates Show COVID-19 Impact on Fertility and Mortality Across the Nation. March 2022. Census Bureau.
https://www.census.gov/library/stories/2022/03/united-states-deaths-spiked-as-covid-19-continued.html. Accessed October 1, 2022.

• Kaba M, Hassan S. Fumbling Towards Repair: A Workbook for Community Accountability Facilitators. AK Press. June 2019. ISBN-13: 9781939202321.

• Karmin A. How Long Does the Fight or Flight Reaction Last? Psych-Central. June 2016.
https://psychcentral.com/blog/anger/2016/06/how-long-does-the-fight-or-flight-reaction-last. Accessed March 22, 2024.

• Karp D, Armour M. The Little Book of Restorative Justice for Colleges and Universities (Second Edition) Repairing Harm and Rebuilding Trust in Response to Student Misconduct. Good Books. September 2019. ISBN: 9781680994681.

• Katella K. Maternal Mortality Is on the Rise: 8 Things To Know. Yale Medicine. May 2023.
https://www.yalemedicine.org/news/maternal-mortality-on-the-rise. Accessed October 20, 2023.

• Kavanagh K. 70% of COVID-19 Cases Transmitted By Children. Infection Control Today®. June 2023.
https://www.infectioncontroltoday.com/view/70-covid-19-cases-trans-mitted-by-children. Accessed October 20, 2023.

• Kesten JM, et al. Changes in the development of opioid tolerance on re-exposure among people who use heroin: A qualitative study. PLoS One. June 2022;17(6):e0269379. doi: 10.1371/journal.pone.0269379. PMID: 35737700.

• Kirzinger, A. Public Knowledge and Attitudes About Sexually Transmitted Infections: KFF Polling and Policy Insights Feb. 2020. Kaiser Family Foundation.
https://www.kff.org/womens-health-policy/issuebrief/public-knowl-edge-and-attitudes-about-sexually-transmittedinfections/#:~:text=child-birth%20(87%25).-,Equally%20large%20shares%20are%20aware%20some%20people%20who%20have%20an,contracting%20the%20STI%20(90%25). Accessed October 14, 2022.

• Klobucista C. U.S. Life Expectancy Is in Decline. Why Aren't Other Countries Suffering the Same Problem? Counsel on Foreign Relations. September 2022.
https://www.cfr.org/in-brief/us-life-expectancydecline-why-arent-other-countries-suffering-same-problem. Accessed October 1, 2022.

• Kordoski M. 'There is hope:' Myrtle Beach mother loses two children to overdose shares her story of loss. WMBF News. September 2023.
https://www.wmbfnews.com/2023/09/26/there-is-hope-myrtle-beachmother-loses-two-children-overdose-shares-her-story-loss/. Accessed October 20, 2023.

• KSAT12, Barajas JP. 'You're not going to make it this time:' Woman says ex-husband shot her then 'hunted' her kids. KSAT12. April 2023.
https://www.ksat.com/news/local/2023/04/18/mother-whosurvived-north-side-shooting-shares-her-story/. Accessed October 20, 2023.

- LAPPA. NALOXONE ACCESS: SUMMARY OF STATE LAWS. LEGISLATIVE ANALYSIS AND PUBLIC POLICY ASSOCIATION . July 2022. https://legislativeanalysis.org/wpcontent/uploads/2022/07/Naloxone-Access-Summary-of-State-Laws.pdf. Accessed October 20, 2023.

- Lawry T. Genetic Code Vs. Zip Code: The Social Determinants Of Health. Forbes. June 2022. https://www.forbes.com/sites/forbestechcouncil/2022/06/13/genetic-code-vs-zip-code-the-socialdeterminants-of-health/?sh=72f1d8e-a581c. Accessed March 22, 2024.

- Leburn-Harris L. Five-Year Trends in US Children's Health and Well-being, 2016-2020. JAMA. March 2022. https://jamanetwork.com/journals/jamapediatrics/fullarticle/2789946 . Accessed October 20, 2023.

- London, L. Red Table Talk: How Women Are Affected By Gun Violence. Red Table Talk. June 2020; S3:E9. https://www.youtube.com/watch?v=vyV721Y_Tt0. Accessed October 20, 2023.

- Long R, Cleveland Manchanda E, Dekker A, Kraynov L, Willson S, Flores P, Samuels E, Rhodes K. Community engagement via restorative justice to build equity-oriented crisis standards of care. Journal of the National Medical Association. August 2022; 114 (4) 377-389. ISSN 0027-9684. https://doi.org/10.1016/j.jnma.2022.02.010.

- Liu P. Achieving Health Equities in Indigenous Peoples in Canada: Learnings Adaptable for Diverse Populations. Circulation. July 2022; 146:153–155. Doi.org/10.1161/CIRCULATIONAHA.122.060773.

- MacMillan A. It's Official: Yoga Helps Depression. ESSENCE. October 2020. https://www.essence.com/lifestyle/health-wellness/yoga-breathing-depression/. Accessed December 9, 2023.

• Mann N. BLACK LONG-COVID SUFFERERS FORM SUPPORT GROUPS AFTER BEING DISMISSED BY DOCTORS. Black Enterprise. August 2022.
https://www.blackenterprise.com/blacklong-covid-sufferers-form-support-groups-after-being-dismissed-by-doctors/. Accessed October 20, 2023.

• Mastroianni B. New Study Finds 47% of LGBTQ People Experience Medical Gaslighting. Healthline. August 2023.
https://www.healthline.com/health-newsnew-study-finds-47-of-lgbtq-people-experiencemedical-gaslighting. Accessed October 20, 2023.

• Maybank A, et. al. Prioritizing Equity: LGBTQ Voices. AMA Center for Health Equity. May 2022.
https://edhub.ama-assn.org/ama-center-health-equity/audio-player/18693555?utm_campaign=alwaysongoogle-paid_ad-lgbtq_dsas_non-brand&gclid=eaiaiqobchmi-5hu07fd-qivxa-tbh2ya8teaayasaaegibypd_bwe#. Accessed August 25, 2022.

• Mayo Clinic Staff (Mayo). Male Breast Cancer. Mayo Clinic. March 2024.
https://www.mayoclinic.org/diseases-conditions/male-breast-cancer/symptoms-causes/syc-20374740. Accessed March 22, 2024.

• McFadden M. The Supreme Court Must Protect Domestic Violence Survivors By Overturning the Rahimi Decision. Teen Vogue. October 2023.
https://www.teenvogue.com/story/supreme-court-protect-domesticviolence-survivors-rahimi-decision. Accessed October 20, 2023.

• McGough M, et al. Child and Teen Firearm Mortality in the U.S. and Peer Countries. KFF. July 2023.
https://www.kff.org/mental-health/issue-brief/child-and-teen-firearm-mortality-in-the-u-s-and-peercountries/. Accessed October 20, 2023.

• McKie R. Revolutionary gene therapy offers hope for untreatable cancers. The Guardian. December 2022.
https://www.theguardian.com/science/2022/dec/11/revolutionary-gene-therapy-offers-hope-untreatablecancers. Accessed October 10, 2023.

• McPhillips D. Nearly 1 in 10 adults in the US has lost a family member to drug overdose, new KFF poll finds. CNN. August 2023. https://www.cnn.com/2023/08/15/health/drug-alcohol-addiction-kffpoll/index.html. Accessed October 10, 2023.

• Million Hearts. "Live to the Beat" Campaign Toolkit. CDC. February 2023.
https://millionhearts.hhs.gov/partners-progress/partners/live-beat-campaign-toolkit.html. Accessed August 11, 2023.

• Mirsky L. Restorative Justice Practices of Native American, First Nation and Other Indigenous People of North America: Part One. IIRP. April 2004. https://www.iirp.edu/news/restorative-justice-practices-ofnative-american-first-nation-and-other-indigenous-people-of-north-america-part-one. Accessed August 11, 2023.

• Moutain State, ProPublica (MtSt/Pro). How Black Communities Become 'Sacrifice Zones' for Industrial Air Pollution. WV Public Broadcasting. December 2021. https://wvpublic.org/how-black-communities-become-sacrifice-zones-for-industrial-air-pollution/. Accessed October 20, 2023.

• Muoio D. Senators Joe Manchin, Marco Rubio introduce bill to make violence, threats against hospital
workers a federal crime. Fierce Healthcare. September 2023. https://www.fiercehealthcare.com/providers/senators-manchin-rubio-introduce-bill-make-violence-threatsagainst-hospital-workers. Accessed October 20, 2023.

• Murphy S, Kochanek K, Xu J, Arias E. Mortality in the United States, 2020. NCHS Data Brief No. 427, December 2021.https://www.cdc.gov/nchs/data/hestat/maternal-mortality/2020/maternal-mortality-rates-2020.htm. Accessed October 20, 2023.

• McEwen B, Stellar E. Stress and the Individual: Mechanisms Leading to Disease. Arch Intern Med. 1993;153(18):2093–2101. doi:10.1001/archinte.1993.00410180039004.

• Mental health America. 4.5 percent identify as lesbian, gay, bisexual, or transgender. 2022. https://mhanational.org/issues/lgbtq-communities-and-mental-health. Accessed October 15, 2023.

• Miller A. A Black doctor died from COVID-19 after she posted a video from her hospital bed saying she was being mistreated: 'This is how Black people get killed.' Business Insider Nederland. December 2020. https://www.businessinsider.nl/a-black-doctor-died-from-covid-19-after-she-posted-a-video-from-herhospital-bed-saying-she-was-being-mistreated-this-is-how-black-people-get-killed/#tbl-emlnt8cjhd-4dkqp6oiskz. Accessed October 20, 2023.

• Minor L. These 5 numbers tell you everything you need to know about racial disparities in health care. Fortune. July 2020. https://fortune.com/2020/07/08/health-care-racism-zip-code-life-expectancy/. Accessed October 20, 2023.

• Montagne R. Israel Kamakawiwo'ole: The Voice Of Hawaii NPR. March 2011. https://www.npr.org/2010/12/06/131812500/israel-kamakawiwo-ole-the-voice-of-hawaii. Accessed October 20, 2023.

• Movement Advancement Project. Where We Call Home: LGBT People in Rural America, Exec summary. MAP. 2019. https://www.lgbtmap.org/file/lgbt-rural-executive-summary.pdf. Accessed December 12, 2023.

• Murthy V. Surgeon General Issues New Advisory About Effects Social Media Use Has on Youth Mental Health. HHS. May 2023. https://www.hhs.gov/about/news/2023/05/23/surgeon-general-issues-newadvisory-about-effects-social-media-use-has-youth-mental-health.html. Accessed October 20, 2023.

• Nagy K. Discharge Instructions for Wound Cares. American Association for the Surgery of Trauma. August 2013. https://www.aast.org/resources-detail/discharge-instructions-wound-cares. Accessed September 22, 2023.

- National Cancer Institute (NCI Common). Common Cancer Types. NCI. March 2023.
https://www.cancer.gov/types/common-cancers Accessed September 24, 2023.

- National Cancer Institute (NCI). What is Cancer? NCI. May 2021.
https://www.cancer.gov/aboutcancer/
understanding/what-is-cancer Accessed October 1, 2022.

- National Center for Chronic Disease Prevention and Health Promotion (NCCDPHP). Cancer. CDC. June
2022. https://www.cdc.gov/chronicdisease/resources/publications/factsheets/cancer.htm. Accessed
September 30, 2022.

- National Center for Health Statistics (CDC Fast Facts). FastStats:Deaths and Mortality. Centers for Disease
Control and Prevention (CDC). January 2022. https://www.cdc.gov/nchs/fastats/deaths.htm .Accessed
July 15, 2022.

- National Center for Health Statistics (CDC FastStats). FastStats: Leading Causes of Death. CDC. 2002.
https://www.cdc.gov/nchs/fastats/leading-causes-of-death.htm Accessed September 22, 2022.

- National Health Services (NHS). Duty of Candor. NHS Resolution. March 2022.
https://resolution.nhs.uk/resources/duty-of-candour-animation/. Accessed October 20, 2023.

- Fraga J. How To Help Kids Overcome Their Fear Of Doctors And Shots. NPR. December 2018.
https://www.npr.org/sections/health-shots/2018/12/29/677505443/
how-to-help-kids-overcome-their-fearof-
doctors-and-shots. Accessed March 22, 2024.

• NASP. Talking to Children About Violence: Tips for Parents and Teachers. 2016.
https://www.nasponline.org/resources-and-publications/resources-and-podcasts/school-safety-andcrisis/school-violence-resources/talking-to-children-about-violence-tips-for-parents-and-teachers. Accessed September 21, 2022.

• National Cancer Institute. Support for Families When a Child Has Cancer. September 2022. National
Institutes of Health. https://www.cancer.gov/about-cancer/coping/caregiver-support/parents. Accessed September 21, 2022.

• National Hospice and Palliative Care Organization (NHPCO). LGBTQ+ Resource Guide. NHPCO. June 2021.
https://www.nhpco.org/wp-content/uploads/LGBTQx_Resource_Guide.pdf. Accessed October 20, 2023.

• National Institute of Mental Health (NIHM). Suicide. NIH. February 2024.
https://www.nimh.nih.gov/health/statistics/suicide. Accessed March 22, 2024.

• National Runaway Safeline (NRS). Here to Listen. Here to Help. NRS. 2024.
https://www.1800runaway.org/. Accessed April 9, 2024.

• Neumann K. Doodle Your Way To Better Mental Health. Forbes. June 2023.
https://www.forbes.com/health/healthy-aging/doodling/. Accessed March 22, 2024.

• National Hospice and Palliative Care Organization (NHPCO L). LGBTQ+ Resource Guide. NHPCO. June 2021.
https://www.google.com/url?sa=t&rct=j&q=&esrc=s&source=web&cd=&ved=2ahUKEwjhv__LgO_5AhUag4kEHbTHAcEQFnoECA0QAQ&url=https%3A%2F%2Fwww.nhpco.org%2Fwpcontent%2Fuploads%2FLGBTQx_Resource_Guide.pdf&usg=AOvVaw3BmvsQEvFwHIObgE9Wr4ql. Accessed August 30, 2022.

• National Hospice and Palliative Care Organization (NHPCO F). NHPCO Facts and Figures Report Shows Growing Number of Hospice Patients. NHPCO. December 2022.
https://www.nhpco.org/nhpco-facts-andfigures-report-shows-growing-number-of-hospicepatients/#:~:text=Growth%20in%20number%20of%20hospice,numbers%20and%20as%20a%20percentage.
Accessed Mach 22, 2024.

• NHPCO. New Facts and Figures Report Shows Changes in Hospice Patient Diagnoses. October 2021.
https://www.nhpco.org/nhpcos-new-facts-and-figures-report-shows-changes-in-hospice-patient-diagnoses/. Accessed September 30, 2022.

• NIDA. Policy Brief: Effective Treatments for Opioid Addiction. NIDA. November 2016.
https://nida.nih.gov/publications/effective-treatments-opioid-addiction. Accessed August 22, 2022.

• NIH. Patient Bill of Rights. U.S. Department of Health and Human Services. May 2021.
https://clinicalcenter.nih.gov/participate/patientinfo/legal/bill_of_rights.html. Accessed October 20, 2023.

• NLHEC. LBGT Voices: Perspectives on Healthcare. Fenway Institute. January 2017.
https://www.lgbtqiahealtheducation.org/video/lgbt-voices-perspectives-on-healthcare/. Accessed October 20, 2023.

• NLHEC. Providing Affirmative Care for Patients with Non-binary Gender Identities. Fenway Institute.
February 2017. https://www.lgbtqiahealtheducation.org/wp-content/uploads/2017/02/Providing-Affirmative-Care-for-People-with-Non-Binary-Gender-Identities.pdf. Accessed October 20, 2023.

• Gramlich F. What the data says about gun deaths in the U.S. Pew Research Center. April 2023.
https://www.pewresearch.org/short-reads/2023/04/26/what-the-data-says-about-gun-deaths-in-the-u-s/. Accessed October 20, 2023.

• O'Bier T. Millions of Americans reported having long COVID. WPTV. September 2023. https://www.wptv.com/millions-of-americans-reported-having-long-covid. Accessed October 20, 2023.

• OPM. Patients' Bill of Rights. U.S. Office of Personnel Management. https://www.opm.gov/healthcareinsurance/healthcare/reference-materials/bill-of-rights/. Accessed October 10, 2023.

• Oyez. "Califano v. Goldfarb." Oyez. www.oyez.org/caes/1976/75-699. Accessed March 24, 2024.

• Panchal N. The Impact of Gun Violence on Children and Adolescents. KFF. February 2024. https://www.kff.org/mental-health/issue-brief/the-impact-of-gun-violence-on-children-and-adolescents/. Accessed October 20, 2023.

• Perkins C. 'We have lost a giant': Ruth Bader Ginsburg (1933–2020). Harvard Law Bulletin. September 2020. https://hls.harvard.edu/today/in-memoriam-ruth-bader-ginsburg/. Accessed October 20, 2023.

• Petrullo J. US Has Highest Infant, Maternal Mortality Rates Despite the Most Health Care Spending. AJMC. January 2023. https://www.ajmc.com/view/us-has-highest-infant-maternal-mortality-rates-despitethe-most-health-care-spending. Accessed October 20, 2023.

• Pew (Pew MAT). The Case for Medication-Assisted Treatment. Pew Charitable Trusts. February 2017. https://www.pewtrusts.org/en/research-and-analysis/fact-sheets/2017/02/the-case-for-medication-assistedtreatment. Accessed October 1, 2022.

• Prachniak C. Creating End-of-Life Documents for Trans Individuals: An Advocates Guide. NationalResource Center on LGBT Aging and Whitman-Walker Health. October 2014. https://www.lgbtagingcenter.org/resources/resource.cfm?r=694. Accessed August 30, 2022.

• Pranis K. Coming Full Circle: Safe Spaces, Learning to "Not Know", and Collective Wisdom. Awakin.org. July 2015.
https://www.awakin.org/v2/calls/218/kay-pranis/.
Accessed August 22, 2022.

• Project Child Safe. Project ChildSafe Safety Kit
https://projectchildsafe.org/safety/get-a-safety-kit/.
Accessed September 21, 2022.

• RAND, Frank L, Concannon T, Patel K. Health Care Resource Allocation Decision making During a Pandemic. RAND Corporation. 2020.
https://www.rand.org/content/dam/rand/pubs/research_reports/
RRA300/RRA326-1/RAND_RRA326-1.pdf. Accessed October 20, 2023.

• Reed J. What you need to know about Covid as new variant rises. BBC. September 2023.
https://www.bbc.com/news/health-66848549. Accessed October 20, 2023.

• Restar A. Gender-affirming care is preventative care. Lancet Reg Health Am. 2023 June;24:100544. doi:10.1016/j.lana.2023.100544. PMID: 37383047.

• Restorative Solutions (Restorative). The Indigenous Origins of Circles and How Non-Natives Learned About Them. Restorative Solutions. October 2017.
https://www.restorativesolutions.us/blog/theindigenous-origins-of-circles-and-how-non-natives-learned-about-them. Accessed August 11, 2023.

• Roberts J, et. al. Justice Ruth Bader Ginsburg. Harv. L. Rev. January 2021; 134 (3). 882-904.

• Russo M, Santarelli D, O'Rourke D. The physiological effects of slow breathing in the healthy human. Breathe (Sheff). December 2017;13(4):298-309. doi: 10.1183/20734735.009817.

• SAEM. Equity in Crisis Standards of Care. Society of Academic Emergency Medicine, September 2020.
https://www.saem.org/docs/default-source/saem-documents/
position-statements/equity-in-crisis-standardsof-care.pdf?s-fvrsn=32bb845f_3. Accessed March 22, 2024.

• SAGE. LGBTQ+ Older People. 2022. https://www.sageusa.org/. Accessed August 30, 2022.

• SAGE (SAGE Get Involved). Get Involved. SAGE. 2023. https://www.sageusa.org/. Accessed October 20, 2023.

• SAMHSA. 988 Suicide & Crisis Lifeline. July 2022. https://www.samhsa.gov/find-help/988. Accessed August 30, 2022.

• SAMHSA. National Helpline. https://www.samhsa.gov/find-help/national-helpline. Accessed August 22, 2022.

• SAMSHA (SAMSHA T). Understanding Child Trauma. NCTSN. 2019. https://store.samhsa.gov/sites/default/files/d7/priv/sma16-4923_0.pdf. Accessed October 20, 2023.

• SAMHSA (SAMHSA M). Medications for Substance Use Disorders. SAMHSA. March 2022. https://www.samhsa.gov/medications-substance-use-disorders. Accessed October 20, 2023.

• Schaechter J. Guns in the Home: Keeping Kids Safe. June 2022. Healthychildren.org. https://www.healthychildren.org/English/safety-prevention/at-home/Pages/Handguns-in-the-Home.aspx. Accessed September 21, 2022.

• Schild D. 'I have admired and loved you almost since the day we met': A resurfaced letter from Ruth Bader Ginsburg's husband illustrates the couple's extraordinary love story. Business Insider. September 2020. https://www.businessinsider.com/ruth-bader-ginsburg-martin-ginsburg-husband-marriage-2020-9. Accessed March 22, 2024.

• Sharman, Z. The Care We Dream Of: Liberatory and Transformative Approaches to LGBTQ+ Health. Arsenal Pulp Press. Vancouver. 2021.

• Shrestha R, Kanchan T, Krishan K. Gunshot Wounds Forensic Pathology. April 2023. https://www.ncbi.nlm.nih.gov/books/NBK556119/. Accessed October 20, 2023.

• Stanford. Teaching LGBTQ+ Health. Stanford Medicine. 2021.
https://mededucation.stanford.edu/courses/teaching-lgbtq-health/.
Accessed August 23, 2022.

• Starting Early. The invisible population — children of the incarcerated. The Burke Foundation. February 2023.
https://newsletter.burkefoundation.org/2023/02/24/the-invisible-population-children-of-theincarcerated/. Accessed October 20, 2023.

• SPLC. NEW ORLEANS HOMEOWNERS STILL IN FINANCIAL STORM 18 YEARS AFTER
KATRINA. August 2023. https://www.splcenter.org/news/2023/08/31/new-orleans-housing-crisis-18-years-hurricane-katrina.
Accessed October 1, 2022.

• Sparks G, et. al. KFF Tracking Poll July 2023: Substance Use Crisis And Accessing Treatment. KFF. August 2023.
https://www.kff.org/other/poll-finding/kff-tracking-poll-july-2023-substance-use-crisis-andaccessing-treatment/. Accessed October 20, 2023.

• Saunders H, Rudowitz R. Will Availability of Over-the-Counter Narcan Increase Access? KFF. September 2023.
https://www.kff.org/policy-watch/will-availability-of-over-the-counter-narcan-increase-access/. Accessed October 20, 2023.

• Slomski A. Thousands of US Youths Cope With the Trauma of Losing Parents to COVID-19. JAMA. November 2021;326(21):2117–2119. doi:10.1001/jama.2021.20846

• Statista. Number of Medicare beneficiaries who received hospice care in the U.S. from 2009 to 2021. Statista. December 2023.
https://www.statista.com/statistics/339851/number-of-hospice-patients-in-the-usper-year/. Accessed October 20, 2023.

• Sterling J, Garcia MM. Cancer screening in the transgender population: a review of current guidelines, best practices, and a proposed care model. Transl Androl Urol. 2020 Dec; 9(6):2771-2785. doi: 10.21037/tau-20-954.

• Stobbe M. Suicides and homicides among young Americans jumped early in the pandemic, study says. AP. June 2023.
https://apnews.com/article/suicide-homicide-children-teens-cdc-39f78929068ba52336b6dccfd6289eb5. Accessed October 20, 2023.

• Survivor Corps. Long COVID FAQs. Survivor Corps. March 2023.
https://www.survivorcorps.com/longcovid-faqs.
Accessed October 20, 2023.

• Swedo E. Prevalence of Adverse Childhood Experiences Among U.S. Adults — Behavioral Risk Factor Surveillance System, 2011–2020. MMWR Morb Mortal Wkly Rep. June 2023;72:707–715. DOI: http://dx.doi.org/10.15585/mmwr.mm7226a2.

• Tannis C, Sale-Shaw J, Lachapelle S, Garland E. Risk Factors and Birth Outcomes of a High-Risk Cohort of Women Served by a Community-Based Prenatal Home Visiting Program. J Community Health Nurs. Jan-Mar 2019;36(1):1-10. doi: 10.1080/07370016.2019.1555318. PMID: 30793959.

• Terao M, Hogan M. When a Child or Adolescent is Diagnosed with Cancer: Words of Support for Parents. Healthychildren.org. September 2020.
https://www.healthychildren.org/English/healthissues/conditions/cancer/Pages/Childhood-Cancer-Coping-With-the-Diagnosis.aspx.
Accessed September 21, 2022.

• Thorne L. The 'highly mutated' COVID variant BA.2.86 — known as Pirola — has landed in Australia. ABC.Net. September 2023.
https://www.abc.net.au/news/2023-09-21/new-covid-strain-variant-pirola-ba-2-86-in-australia-symptoms/102873304.
Accessed January 6, 2024.

• Torre G. First Nations Health Authority in Canada given $8.2 billion and power to set their own course. NIT. April 2023.
https://nit.com.au/16-04-2023/5611/first-nations-health-authority-in-canada-given-82-billion-and-power-to-set-their-own-course.
Accessed December 11, 2023.

• Totenberg N. Justice Ruth Bader Ginsburg, Champion Of Gender Equality, Dies At 87. NPR. September 2020.
https://www.npr.org/2020/09/18/100306972/justice-ruth-bader-gins-burg-champion-of-genderequality-dies-at-87.
Accessed October 10, 2023.

• Center for Labor Education & Research University of Hawaii (UH). Hawaii Law of The Aloha Spirit. UH.
https://www.hawaii.edu/uhwo/clear/home/lawaloha.html.
Accessed March 22, 2024.

• USA Facts. Children are dying at the fastest rate in 13 years. CDC. June 2023.
https://usafacts.org/dataprojects/child-death. Accessed October 20, 2023.

• U.S. Census Bureau (US Census). U.S. and World Population Clock. USCB. July 2022.
https://www.census.gov/popclock/. Accessed January 6, 2024.

• U.S. Department of Justice (USDJ). ADA Business BRIEF: Communicating with People Who Are Deaf or Hard of Hearing in Hospital Settings. USDJ. October 2003.
https://archive.ada.gov/hospcombr.htm#:~:text=Hospitals%20can-not%20charge%20patients%20or,rather%20than%20a%20standard%20telephone. Accessed March 22, 2024.

• van Doremalen N, et. al. Aerosol and Surface Stability of SARS-CoV-2 as Compared with SARS-CoV-1. N Engl J Med 2020; 382:1564-1567. DOI: 10.1056/NEJMc2004973.

• Wailling J, Marshall, C., Wilkinson, J. Hearing and responding to the stories of survivors of surgical mesh: Nga korero a nga morehu – he urupare (A report for the Ministry of Health). The Diana Unwin Chair in Restorative Justice, Victoria University of Wellington December 2019.

• Wallace M. Homicide During Pregnancy and the Postpartum Period in the United States, 2018-2019. Obstet Gynecol. February 2022;139(2):347. PMID: 34619735.

• Webster R, Adelson J. The Federal Program to Rebuild After Hurricane Katrina Shortchanged the Poor. New Data Proves It. December 2022. https://www.propublica.org/article/how-louisiana-road-homeprogram-shortchanged-poor-residents. Accessed October 1, 2022.

• World Health Organization (WHO C). Advice for the Public: Coronavirus Disease (COVID-19). WHO. 2022. https://www.who.int/emergencies/diseases/novel-coronavirus-2019/advice-for-public. Accessed September 28, 2022.

• World Health Organization (WHO Cancer). Cancer. 2022. https://www.who.int/healthtopics/cancer#tab=tab_1. Accessed September 24, 2022.

• World Health Organization (WHO D). WHO COVID-19 Dashboard. 2023. WHO. https://data.who.int/dashboards/covid19/cases?n=c. Accessed October 16, 2023.

• World Health Organization (WHO Prev). Preventing cancer. WHO. 2023. https://www.who.int/activities/preventing-cancer. Accessed March 22, 2024.

• World Health Organization (WHO 10). The top 10 causes of death. WHO. December 2020. https://www.who.int/news-room/fact-sheets/detail/the-top-10-causes-of-death. Accessed July 15, 2022.

• Worldmeter. United States Population (Live). Worldmeter. July 2023. https://www.worldometers.info/world-population/us-population/. Accessed January 6, 2024.

• World Population Review (WPR). Burial Laws by State 2024. World Population Review. 2024.
https://worldpopulationreview.com/state-rankings/burial-laws-by-state. Accessed March 22, 2024.

• Yazzie CJR (Yazzie CJ). About Peacemaking -Robert Yazzie. Indigenous Peacekeeping Initiative. September 2016.
https://peacemaking.narf.org/2015/10/robert-yazzie/. Accessed December 11, 2023.

• Yazzie CJR (Yazzie). Life Comes From It: Navajo justice. Context.org/ Context Institute. June 2016.
https://www.dailygood.org/story/1327/life-comes-from-it-navajo-justice-chief-justice-robert-yazzie/. Accessed December 11, 2023.

• YoungMinds. Racism and mental health. YoungMinds. 2021.
https://www.youngminds.org.uk/youngperson/coping-with-life/racism-and-mental-health/#Howcanexperiencingracismaffectmymentalhealth. Accessed December 11, 2023.